MENTAL HEALTH GUIDES

UNDERSTANDING ADHD

by Doris Edwards

BrightPoint Press

San Diego, CA

BrightPoint Press

an imprint of ReferencePoint Press, Inc.
Printed in the United States

For more information, contact:
BrightPoint Press
PO Box 27779
San Diego, CA 92198
www.BrightPointPress.com

Content Consultant: Elizabeth Lefler, PhD, Licensed Psychologist, Associate Professor of Psychology, University of Northern Iowa

LIBRARY OF CONGRESS CATALOGING-IN-PUBLICATION DATA

Names: Edwards, Doris, author.
Title: Understanding ADHD / Doris Edwards.
Description: San Diego, CA : BrightPoint Press, [2022] | Series: Mental health guides | Includes bibliographical references and index. | Audience: Grades 7-9
Identifiers: LCCN 2021005256 (print) | LCCN 2021005257 (eBook) | ISBN 9781678201364 (hardcover) | ISBN 9781678201371 (eBook)
Subjects: LCSH: Attention-deficit hyperactivity disorder. | Attention-deficit-disordered children. | Attention-deficit hyperactivity disorder--Treatment. | Attention-deficit-disordered children--Treatment.
Classification: LCC RJ506.H9 E39 2022 (print) | LCC RJ506.H9 (eBook) |
DDC 618.92/8589--dc23
LC record available at https://lccn.loc.gov/2021005256
LC eBook record available at https://lccn.loc.gov/2021005257

AT A GLANCE

- Attention deficit hyperactivity disorder (ADHD) is one of the most common neurodevelopmental disorders.
- ADHD is usually inherited. It can also be caused by a brain injury or exposure to environmental toxins.
- ADHD is usually diagnosed in childhood and can last into adulthood.
- There are three presentations of ADHD: predominantly inattentive, predominantly hyperactive-impulsive, and combined.
- Common symptoms of inattention include forgetfulness and lack of focus.
- Common symptoms of hyperactivity and impulsivity include fidgety behavior and impatience.

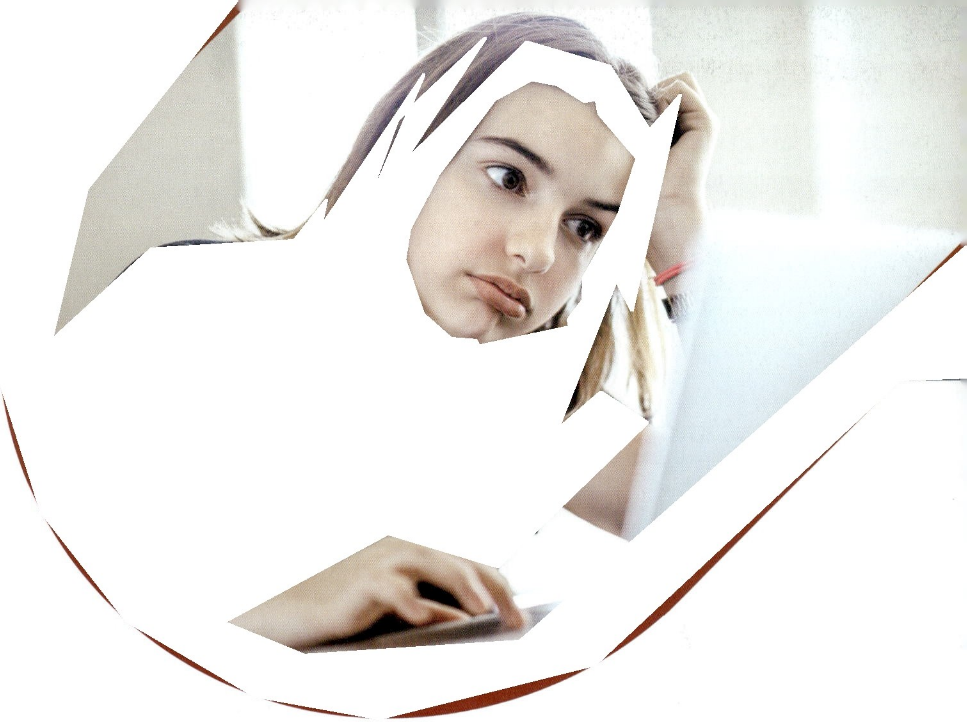

- Early symptoms of ADHD usually appear between the ages of three and six years. These symptoms may not cause problems until later.
- Approximately 5.9 percent of children and teens in the United States have ADHD.
- Boys are two to three times more likely to be diagnosed with ADHD than girls.
- The three main treatments for ADHD are behavioral therapy, classroom help, and medication.

AN OLYMPIC SUPERSTAR WITH GOLD-MEDAL FOCUS

Simone Biles is the most decorated gymnast of all time. She is known for performing difficult gymnastic skills. Biles had received a combination of thirty World Championship and Olympic medals by 2019. By that year she had won nineteen

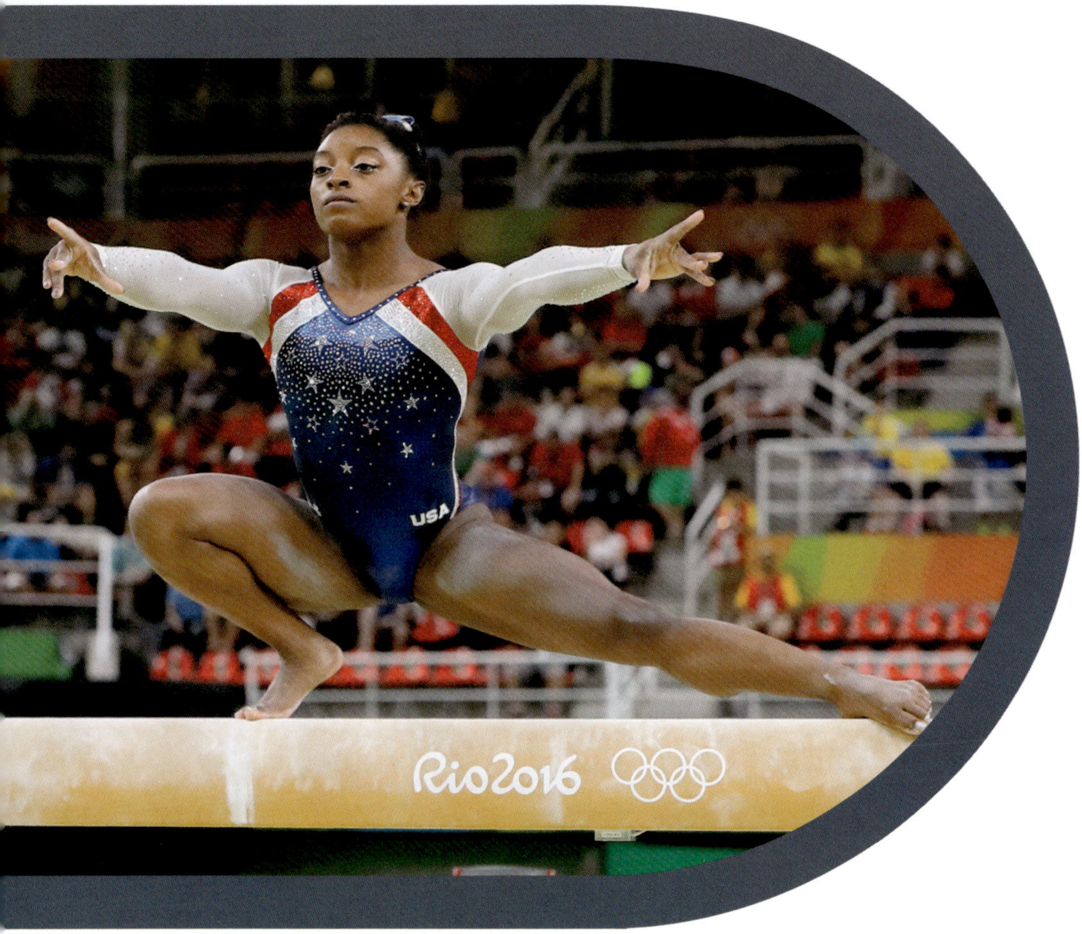

Simone Biles is an Olympic gymnast. She has spoken about her ADHD diagnosis.

gold, three silver, and three bronze World medals. That's the most in gymnastic history. She is also the first woman to win five world all-around titles.

Biles's path to stardom wasn't easy. Her medical records were stolen in 2016. The records showed Biles was taking a stimulant. This is a type of drug that improves some of the brain's processes. A group of Russian hackers leaked this information. They accused Biles of using a drug to improve her performance.

But Biles wasn't cheating. She had taken a medication called Ritalin for years to treat a health problem. The Olympic Committee knew Biles was taking Ritalin. The committee confirmed that she had been allowed to continue her medication

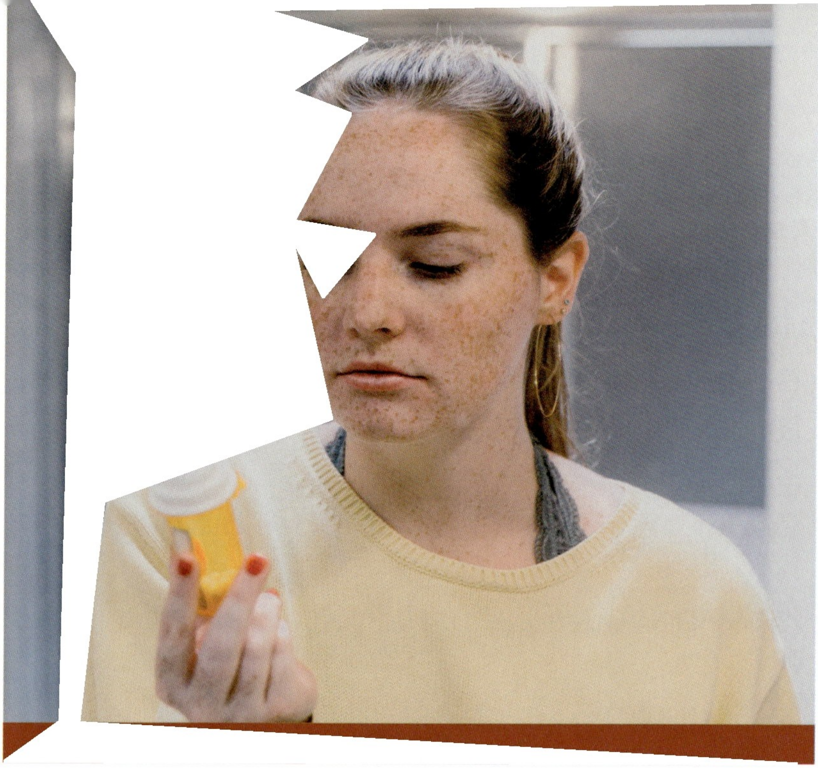

Certain types of medication can help treat ADHD.

while competing. Biles also posted an explanation on Twitter. “I have ADHD and I have taken medicine for it since I was a kid,” she tweeted. “Please know, I believe in clean sport, have always followed the rules, . . . as fair play is critical to sport and is very important to me.”[1]

ABOUT ADHD

ADHD, or attention deficit hyperactivity disorder, is a mental and behavioral health condition. It affects a person's thinking and behavior. ADHD is usually diagnosed during childhood and can last into adulthood. The disorder affects approximately 5.9 percent of children and teens in the United States.

Diagnosing ADHD can be tricky. But there are signs to look for, such as fidgeting or an inability to focus. These behaviors cause problems. A child with ADHD struggles more with these behaviors than a child without ADHD. Untreated ADHD

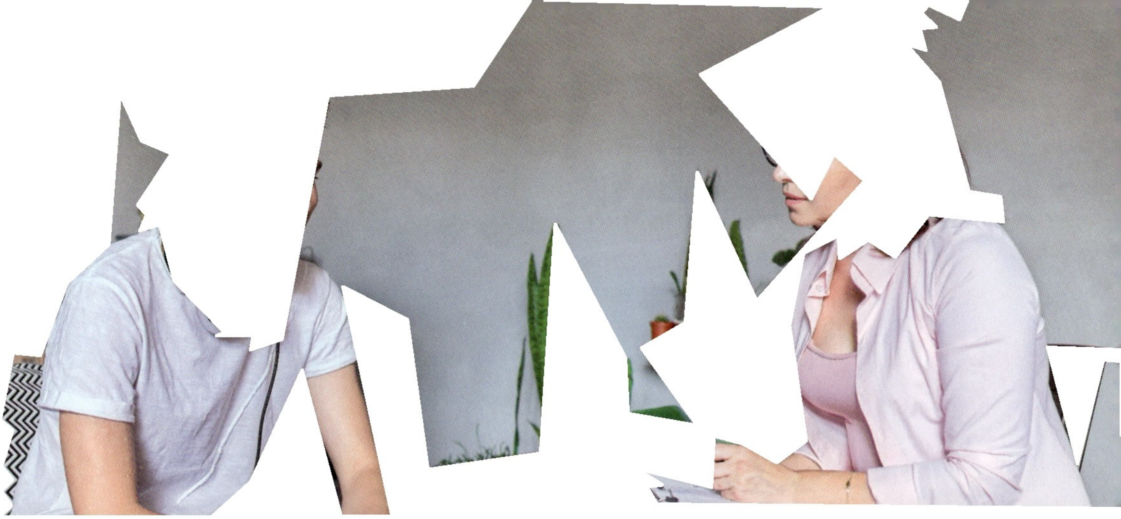

Mental health professionals are able to diagnose ADHD.

can get in the way of schoolwork or daily chores. It can strain relationships with family and friends.

But there are treatments for ADHD. Many people with the condition go on to achieve great success. Simone Biles is a perfect example. “Having ADHD, and taking medicine for it is nothing to be ashamed of,” she tweeted.[2]

CHAPTER ONE

WHAT IS ADHD?

ADHD is one of the most common mental health conditions. It is a neurodevelopmental disorder. This means it begins to affect the brain early in a person's life.

ADHD impacts people in different ways. One person with ADHD might find it difficult to pay attention. Another might show **impulsive** behavior. She might

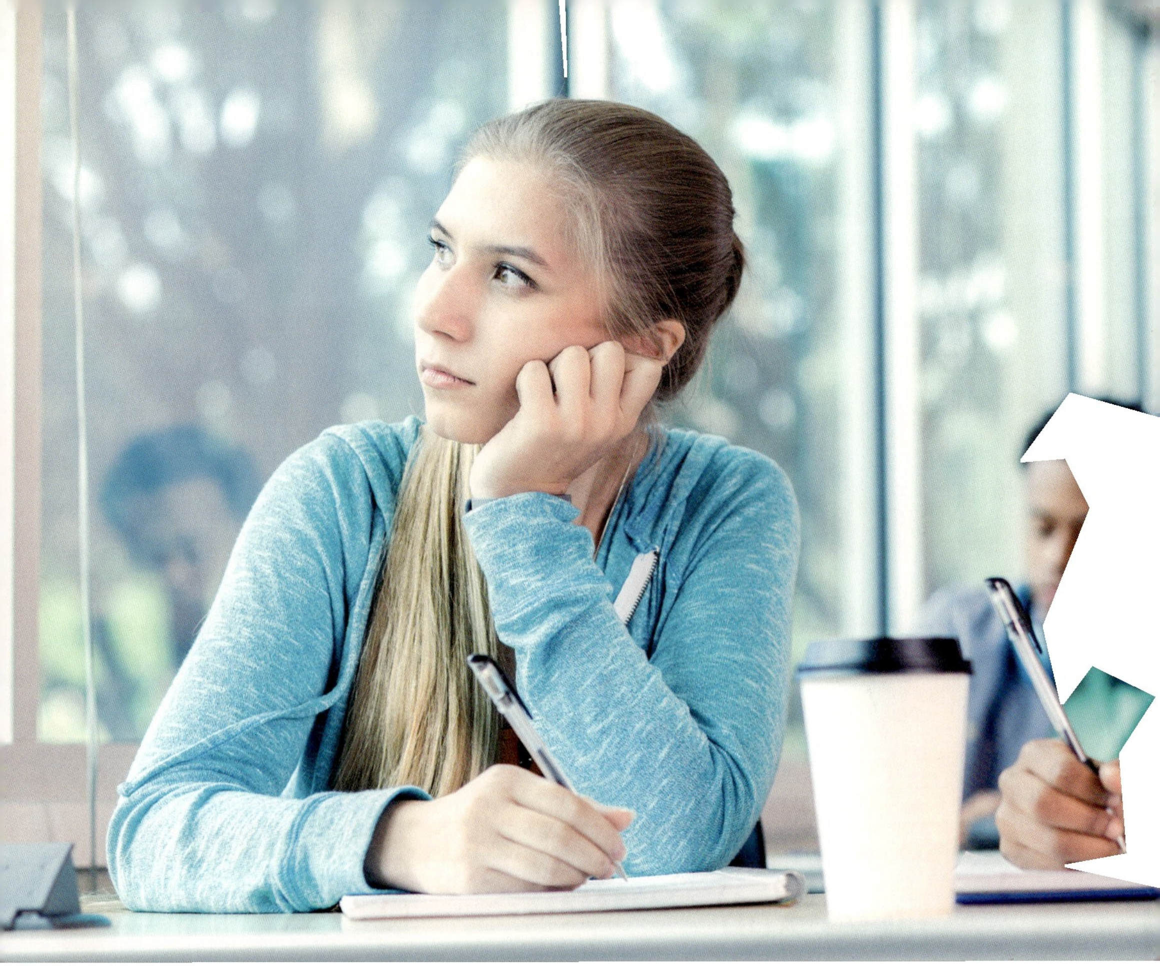

A student with ADHD may have a difficult time paying attention in class.

make decisions without thinking about the consequences. A different person with ADHD could act hyper. He might have difficulty sitting still for long periods of time.

People with ADHD may experience these behaviors at different times in their lives.

According to the American Psychiatric Association, there are three presentations of ADHD. They are predominantly inattentive, predominantly hyperactive-impulsive, and

ADHD VS. ADD

Doctors use the *Diagnostic and Statistical Manual of Mental Disorders* (*DSM-5*) to diagnose mental health conditions. In the past, the book included attention deficit disorder (ADD). This term described people who had problems paying attention but were not hyperactive. The *DSM* was updated in 2013. The term *ADD* was removed. ADD is no longer a diagnosis. Today, these patients are described as having predominantly inattentive ADHD.

combined. There are two types of ADHD **symptoms**. One is inattention. The other is hyperactivity and impulsivity.

PREDOMINANTLY INATTENTIVE PRESENTATION

People with predominantly inattentive ADHD have trouble focusing. They are easily distracted. They also have a hard time finishing tasks.

For example, a sixth grader without ADHD might have a typical morning routine. She gets up in the morning and eats breakfast. Then she gets dressed. She brushes her teeth before leaving to catch

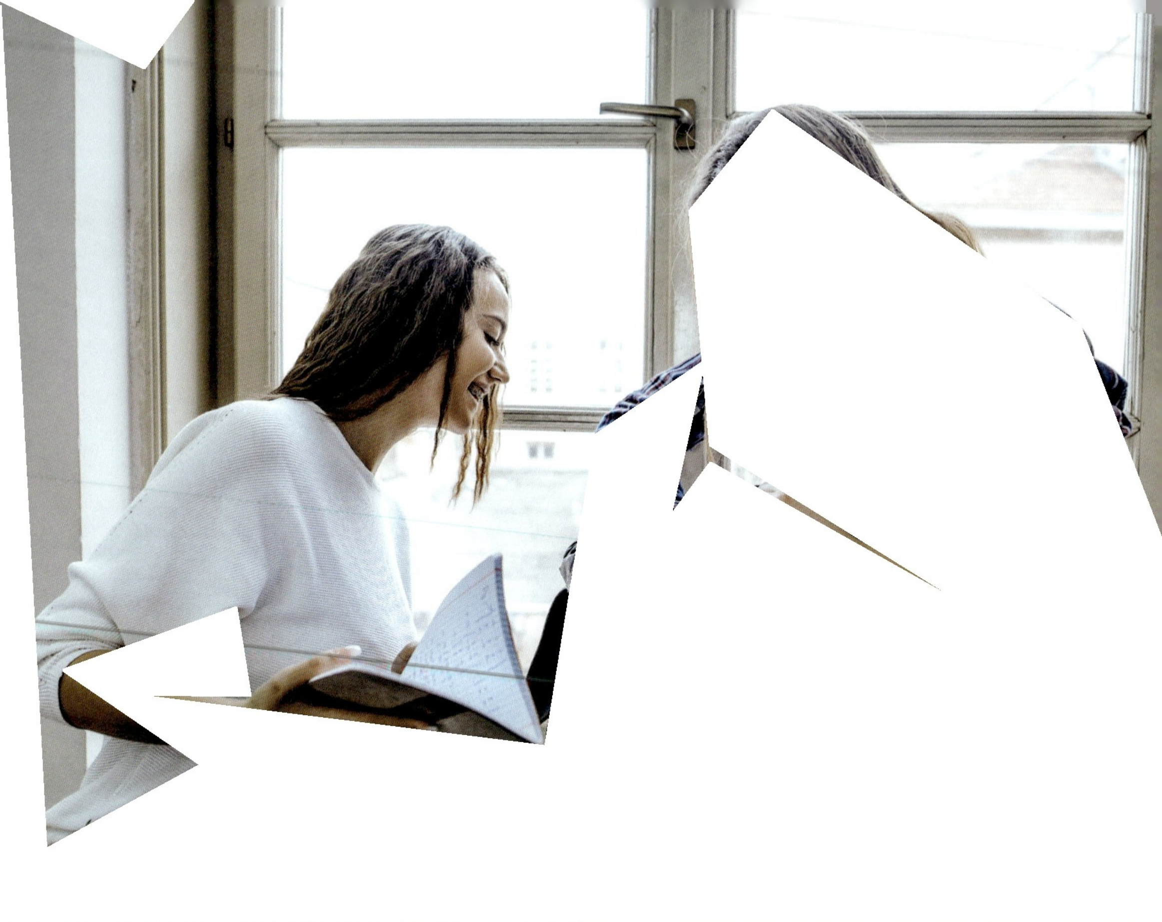

Someone with predominantly inattentive ADHD may be forgetful or misplace things.

the school bus. She usually remembers all of her homework.

A person with predominantly inattentive ADHD might have the same daily routine. But he struggles when the routine is interrupted. He might forget to brush his teeth because he started focusing on what to wear. Or he might get distracted by his music. The shift in attention causes him to forget to pack his math book before leaving for the bus.

PREDOMINANTLY HYPERACTIVE-IMPULSIVE PRESENTATION

The second kind of ADHD is predominantly hyperactive-impulsive. People with this kind of ADHD have difficulty staying still. They feel restless. They may interrupt others. Sometimes they act without thinking things through.

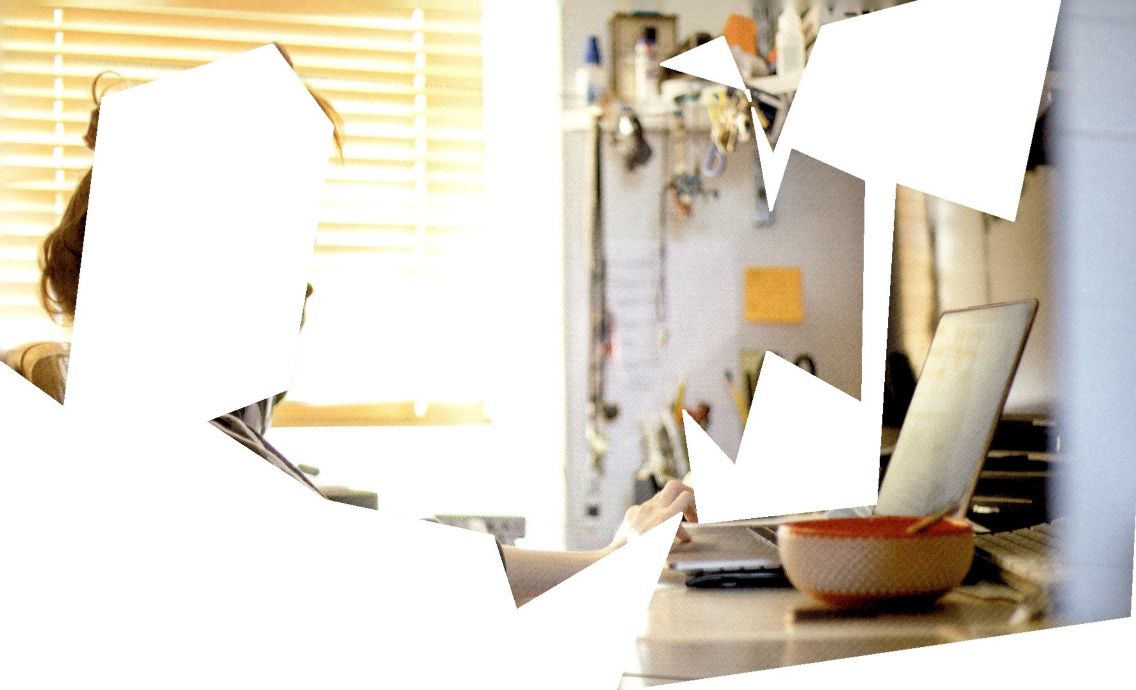

Fidgeting is a common behavior of someone with predominantly hyperactive-impulsive ADHD.

For example, a student without ADHD might get bored during a history lesson. But he'd stay in his seat throughout the entire period. He'd raise his hand before asking a question. At recess, he'd patiently wait for his turn during a game of softball. When not at bat, he might talk to his friends.

A kid with predominantly hyperactive-impulsive ADHD would do things differently. She might get up often during class. She would yell out the answers to the teacher's questions. During softball she might do jumping jacks. This may cause her to miss her turn to bat.

Clinical **psychologist** Dr. David Anderson has studied children with this kind of ADHD. "You've got a kid who's more likely to look for the short-term payoff than long-term payoffs," he says. "You've got a kid who doesn't want to wait . . . who's quickly distractable."[3]

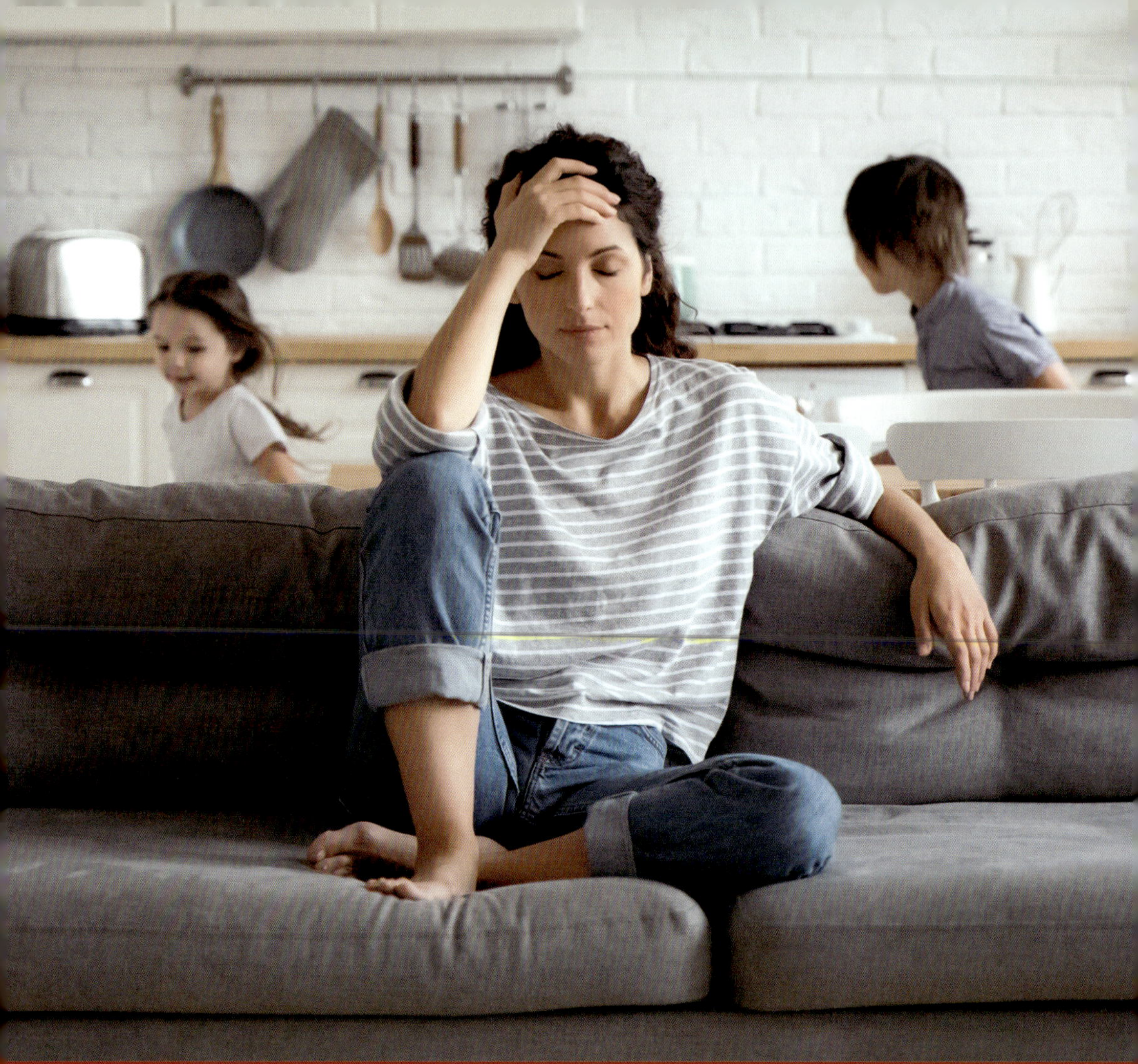

Hyperactivity in young kids can be stressful for parents.

COMBINED PRESENTATION

The third kind of ADHD is combined hyperactive-impulsive and inattentive. It is the most common type. People with this kind of ADHD show both inattentive and hyperactive symptoms. These include difficulty paying attention, hurried behavior, and high levels of energy.

In all three of these presentations, symptoms can change over time. It is possible for someone to start out with one kind of ADHD, then change to another. People can show different symptoms in different situations.

CAUSES

Doctors think ADHD is caused by a combination of factors. One is a person's genes. Genes are instructions that represent certain traits. For example, genes determine a person's eye color. They are passed from parent to child. ADHD runs in families. A child could inherit genes that may cause ADHD.

MYTHS BUSTED

Some people think things like eating too much sugar or playing too many video games cause ADHD. Others claim that doing these things can cause temporary hyperactivity. These are myths. Studies have shown excess sugar, video games, and TV do not cause ADHD or even short-term hyperactivity. Kids with ADHD might have a hard time stopping a TV binge. But their disorder is not getting worse.

Another factor is the environment. Exposure to lead paint has been linked with ADHD in children. Being around **pesticides** at an early age can increase the risk of ADHD. Premature birth and low birth weight are also linked to ADHD.

Scientists have found brain differences in people with ADHD. Some parts of the brain are smaller in children with ADHD. People with ADHD also produce less norepinephrine. These lower levels make it difficult to pay attention. Norepinephrine is a neurotransmitter. Neurotransmitters are chemicals that help send messages

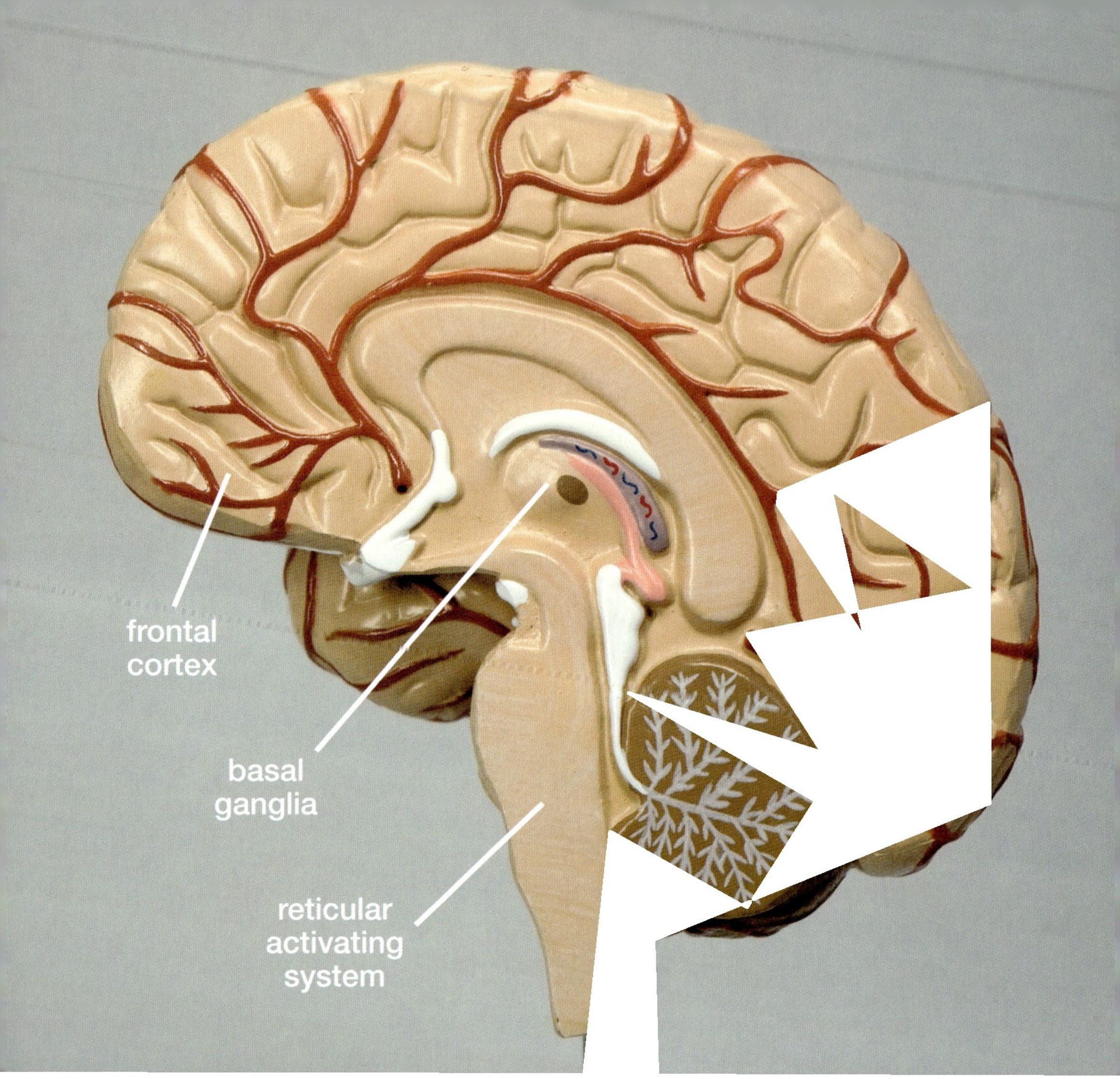

Some parts of the brain are very important for planning and focus.

within the brain. They also help the brain communicate with the rest of the body.

Having less norepinephrine weakens activity in some areas of the brain. This causes problems because areas of the brain interact with each other. For example, the frontal cortex helps with organization. An issue here makes it difficult to plan or make decisions. The limbic system is also impacted. It manages emotion and attention. The basal ganglia and reticular activating system help with focus. Low levels of norepinephrine affect these brain regions too. This results in behaviors such as inattention and impulsivity.

CHAPTER TWO

HOW DOES ADHD AFFECT PEOPLE?

It is normal for young children to act hyper. A lot of teens have trouble focusing too. But some kids and teens never grow out of this behavior. For people with ADHD, these issues are extreme.

ADHD symptoms typically first appear between the ages of three and six.

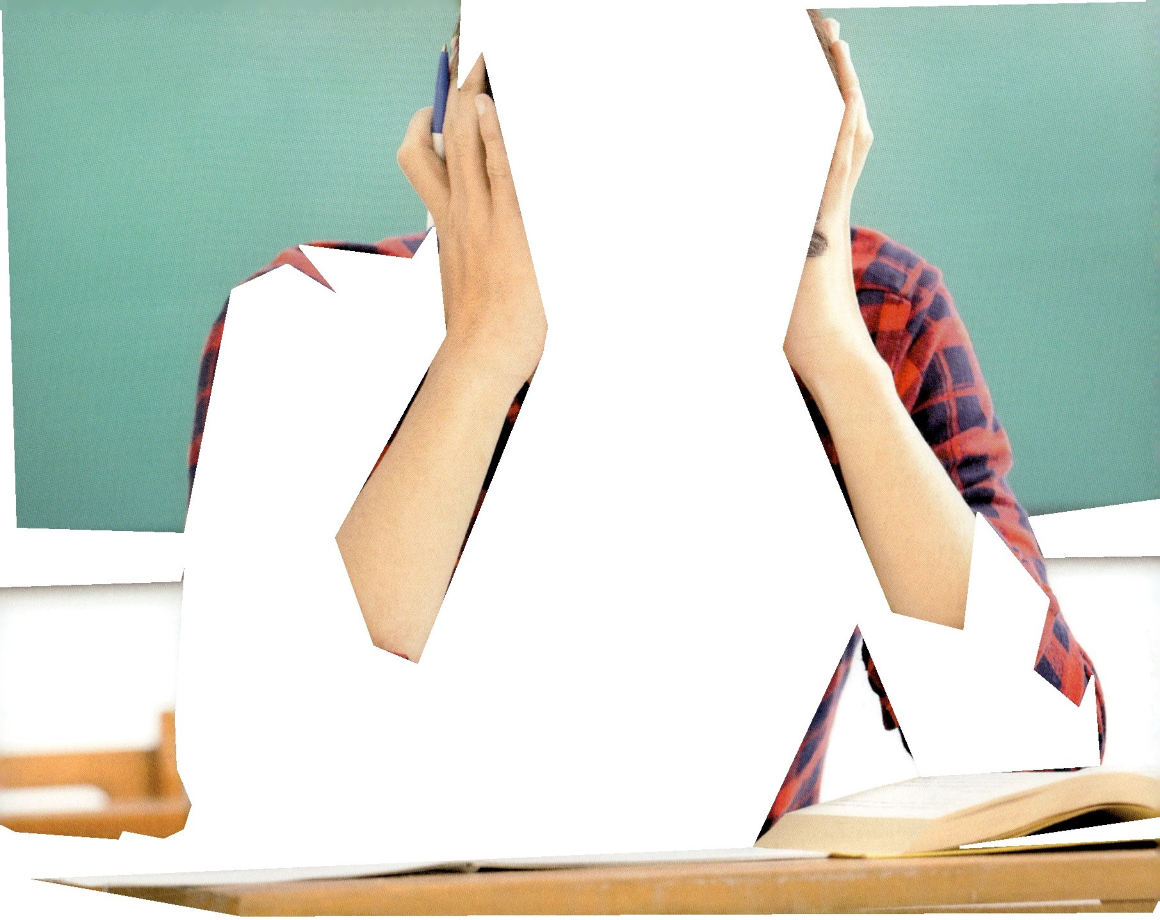

ADHD can cause difficulties in school.

They may change over time and can also last into adulthood. These symptoms cause behaviors that get in the way of daily life. These behaviors can vary from person to person. They may cause someone to get

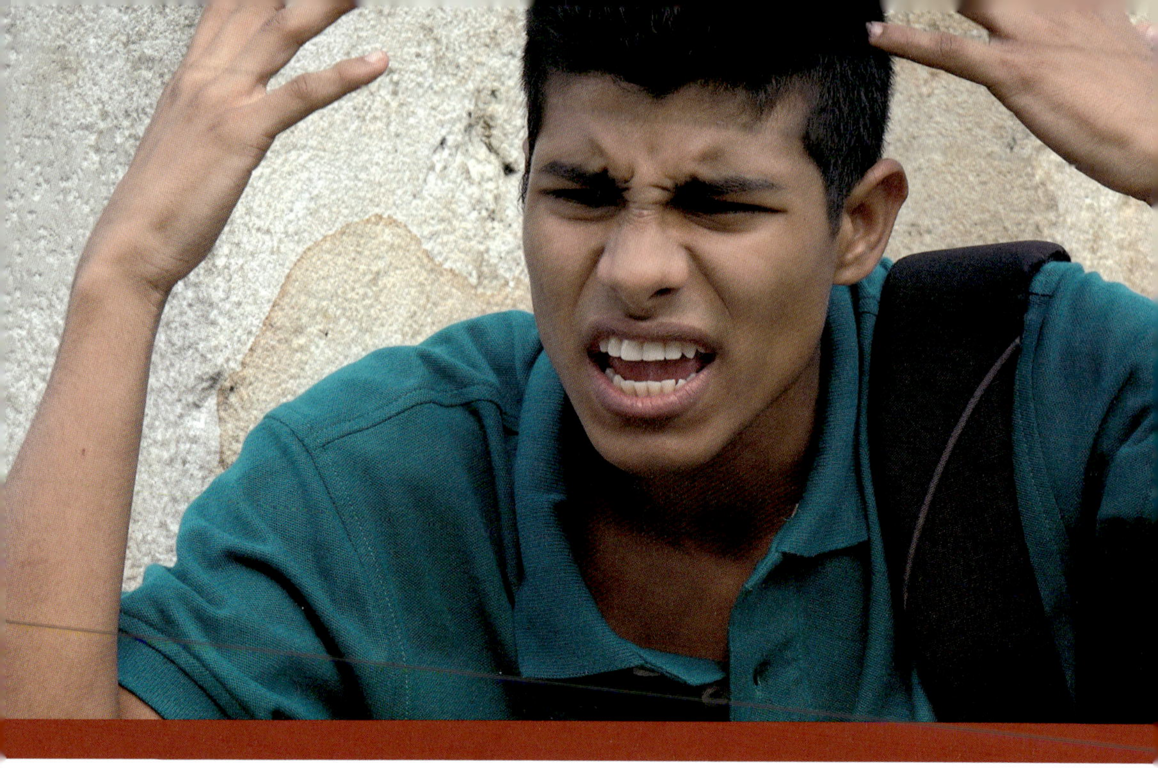

Someone with ADHD may have a hard time controlling his temper.

lower grades than he or she is capable of. A person may have difficulties controlling his or her emotions. He or she may struggle to make friends.

ADHD symptoms can be mild, moderate, or severe. They differ from person to person. And the symptoms can be similar to symptoms of other mental health conditions. This can make ADHD difficult to diagnose. But there are certain signs that doctors look for.

INATTENTION SYMPTOMS OF ADHD

People with inattention symptoms have trouble paying attention to details. Focusing on one task at a time can be tricky. Daydreaming is common.

Another characteristic of inattention is having poor organizational skills. This can make it difficult to complete projects. Some people are easily distracted. Others are forgetful. They misplace things such as

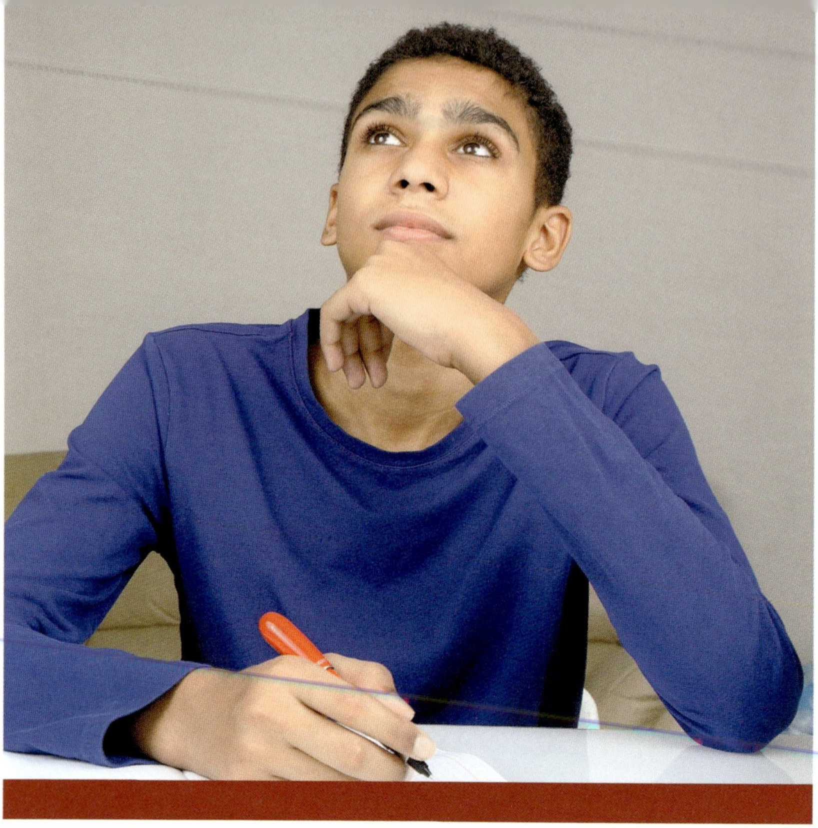

Difficulty staying focused is an inattention symptom of ADHD.

their keys and wallet. These behaviors are common for those with inattentive ADHD.

HYPERACTIVITY AND IMPULSIVITY SYMPTOMS OF ADHD

One of the telltale signs of hyperactive-impulsive ADHD is fidgeting. For example, a student with this kind of ADHD might tap her fingers on her desk constantly. Or she may jiggle her foot repeatedly during class.

Out-of-place behavior is also common. For example, a second grader with hyperactive-impulsive ADHD might climb on tables in the cafeteria. Or he may have difficulty participating in activities quietly. He may make frequent comments while watching a movie.

People who have hyperactive-impulsive symptoms are usually in motion. Some talk nonstop or interrupt conversations. Others have trouble waiting their turn. Many people

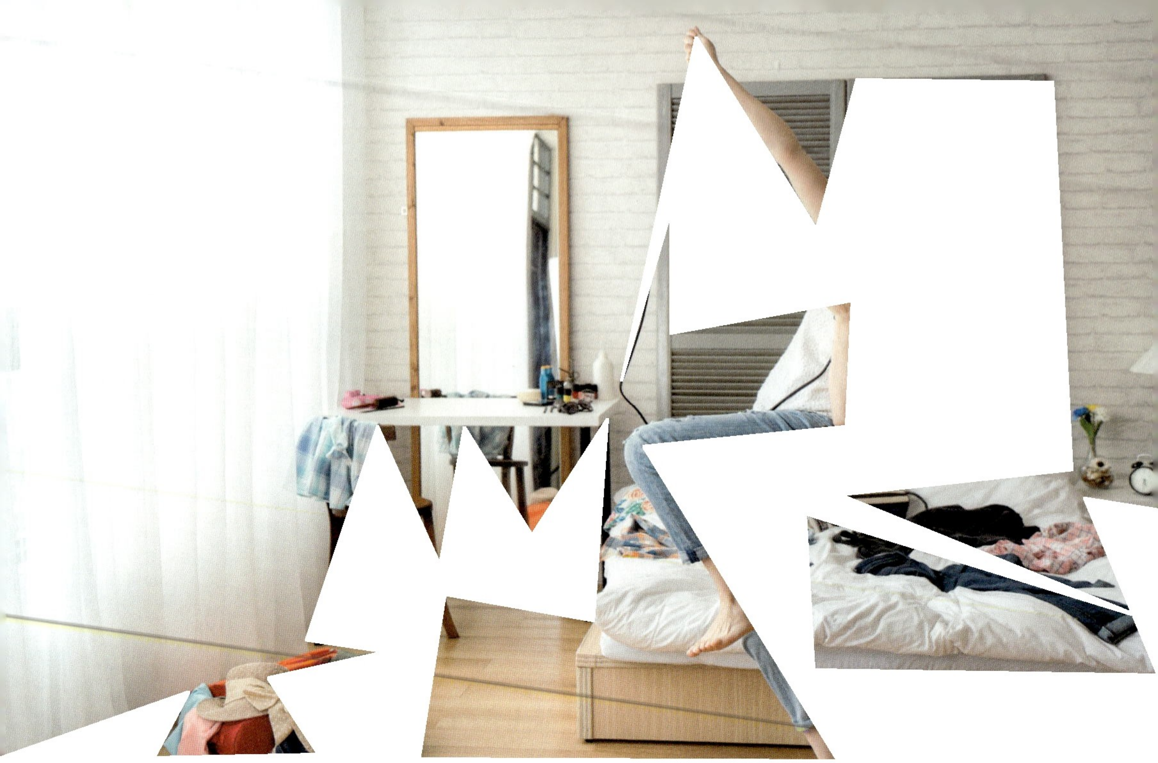

Someone with many hyperactive and impulsive symptoms of ADHD finds it hard to stay still.

with this type of ADHD have a hard time staying in their seats.

A DIAGNOSIS

There isn't a perfect test to figure out if a patient has ADHD. But there are steps to receiving an accurate diagnosis. Most patients see a primary care doctor first. They may be referred to an ADHD specialist or a child psychologist.

Before the appointment, the child's parent or guardian is usually given a questionnaire to fill out. It asks questions about the patient's behavior over the past six months. The child's teachers may also fill out forms to describe his or her behavior at school. A guidance counselor can also provide feedback.

The mental health professional will then gather more information about the patient's symptoms during the appointment. They also might do additional testing. Inattention and hyperactivity-impulsivity each have nine symptoms. A child must show six of one type to be diagnosed. Children with combined ADHD show symptoms of inattention and hyperactivity-impulsivity. They have at least six symptoms of both types. People seventeen and older need five symptoms of one type for a diagnosis.

The average age for an ADHD diagnosis is seven years old. But people may receive an ADHD diagnosis later in life too. In this case, they must have shown symptoms before age twelve to receive the diagnosis.

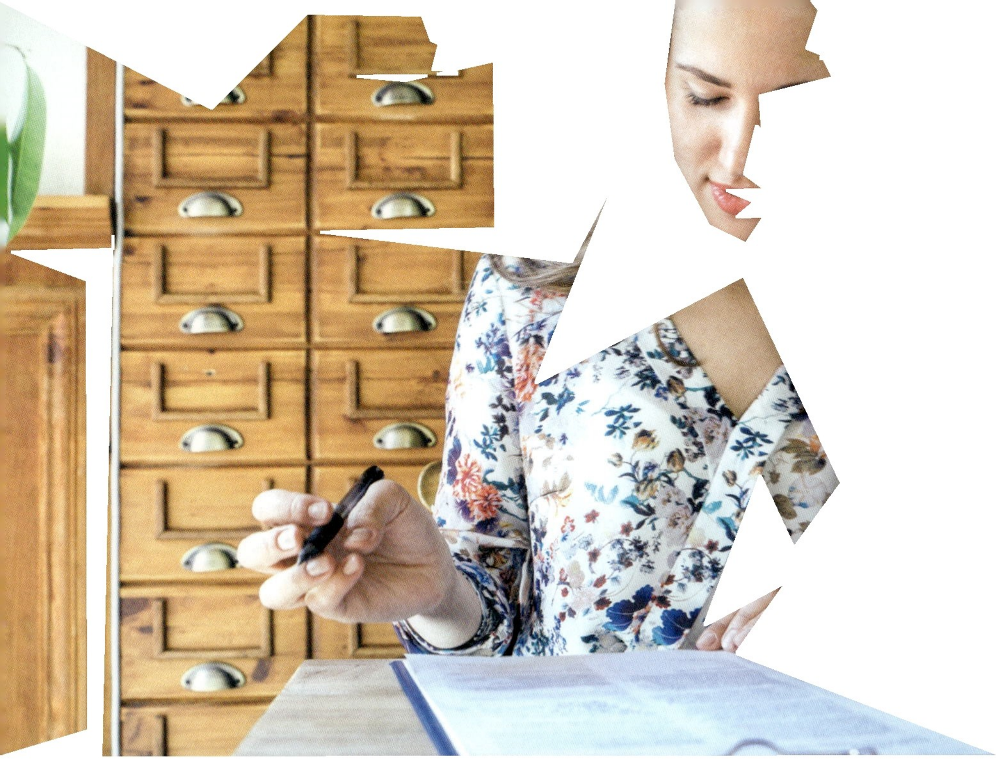

A child psychologist may ask teachers and parents to describe a child's behavior.

Symptoms must be present in multiple settings, such as at school and at home.

MULTIPLE CONDITIONS

Children and Adults with Attention Deficit Hyperactivity Disorder (CHADD) provides support for people with ADHD. It found that more than two-thirds of children with ADHD have another mental health condition. This can make ADHD difficult to diagnose. Some conditions include anxiety, depression, and learning disorders. More than half of those

ADHD RATING SCALE

ADHD can be diagnosed only by a mental health professional. But there is a rating scale that people can use before seeing a doctor. The NICHQ Vanderbilt Assessment Scale is used to assess behaviors of children ages six to twelve. Parents and teachers fill out the rating scale. They rate how often the child shows certain behaviors. If behaviors occur frequently, a person could have ADHD. The parent may want to schedule an appointment to receive a formal diagnosis.

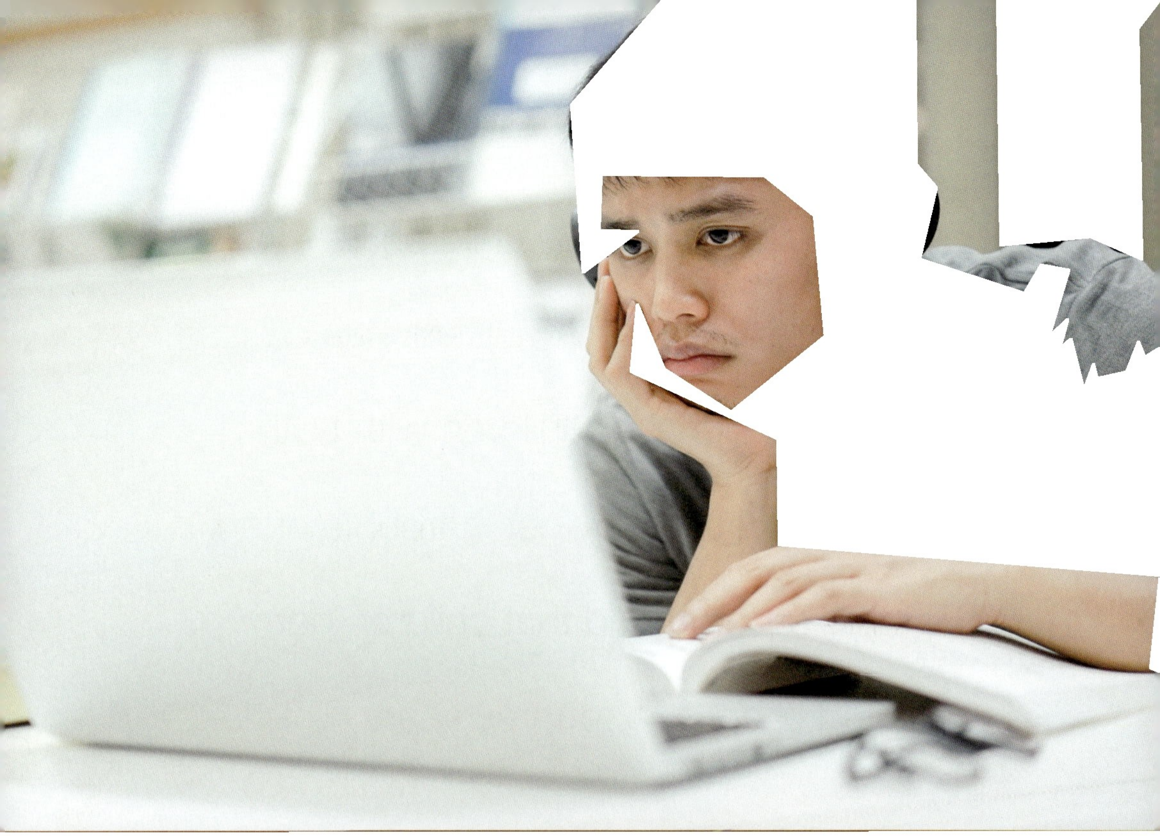

Many people with ADHD also have dyslexia. This leads to struggles with reading.

with ADHD have dyslexia. This causes trouble with reading. About 40 percent of people with ADHD show other behavior problems. They have oppositional defiant disorder (ODD) or conduct disorder. These are patterns of **hostile** behavior toward authority figures. These children have a hard time controlling their impulses. This causes them to misbehave. Children with both ADHD and ODD may get in trouble often. Doctors recommend that children get retested every two to three years. This helps

ODD AND CONDUCT DISORDER

Kids with ODD or conduct disorder may be disobedient. They have trouble controlling their impulses. But the disorders are different. Those with ODD get angry easily. They may argue with parents and teachers. Kids with conduct disorder show more extreme behaviors. They may bully others and start fights. They may steal or break other laws.

determine whether behavior is caused by ADHD or another condition.

STIGMA

Even before a diagnosis, people with ADHD may experience stigma. This stigma may come from other people. Incorrect beliefs about ADHD may cause the person with ADHD to feel ashamed. Stigma can also come from oneself.

People who do not have ADHD may have a negative view of ADHD behavior. They may not understand ADHD symptoms. This can be harmful to people with ADHD. Teachers and adults may have a negative view of a girl with hyperactive behavior. They may treat her differently than a boy with similar symptoms. Someone without ADHD may think ADHD behavior is childish. Or he may think a person with ADHD is lazy because she has trouble paying attention.

Someone with ADHD may begin to believe what others say about his behavior. He may feel ashamed of his diagnosis. He may believe he cannot succeed. This can result in low self-esteem.

But these negative attitudes are untrue. ADHD is a medical condition. People cannot control their ADHD symptoms.

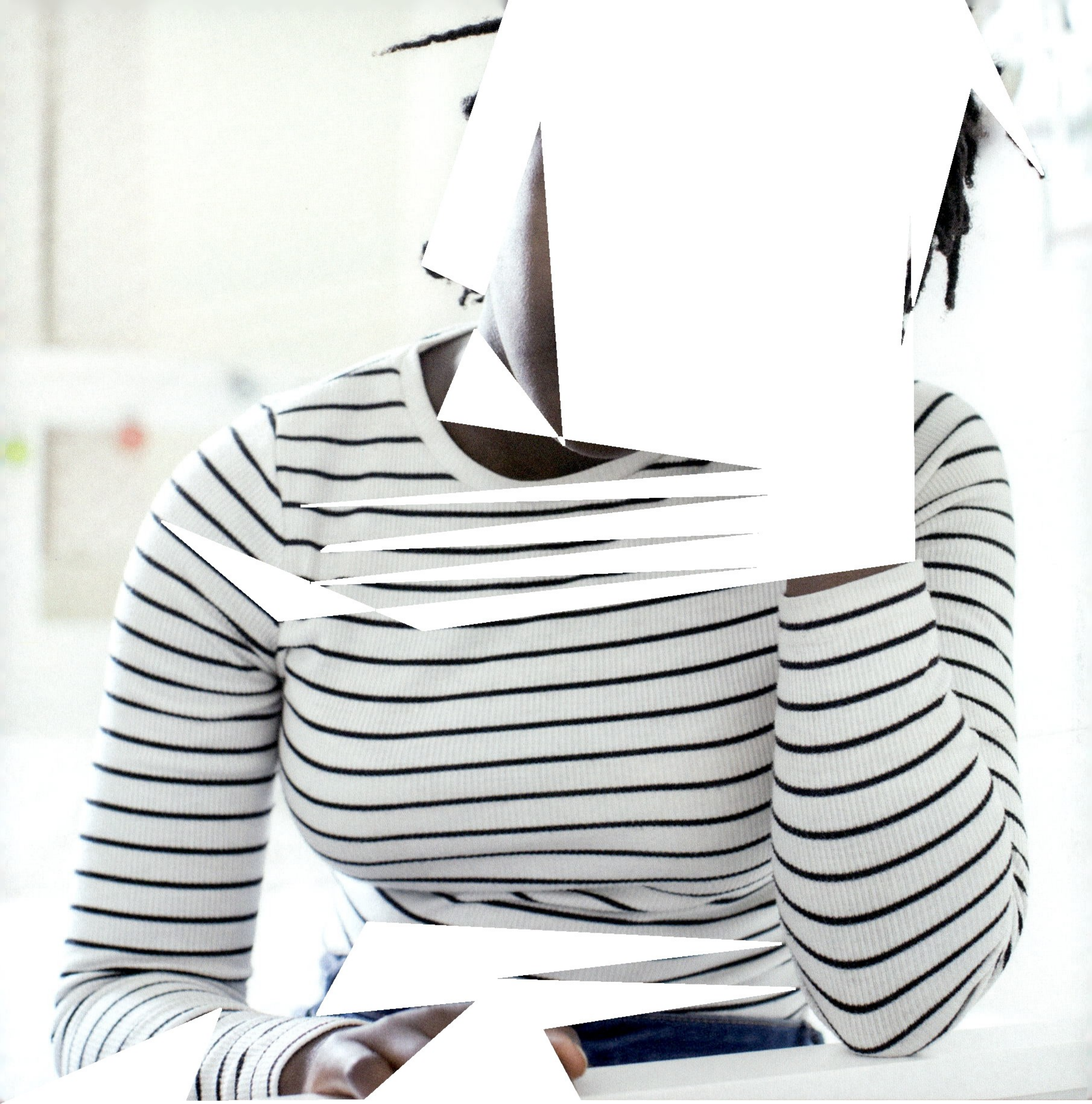

Stigma about ADHD can lower self-esteem and cause feelings of shame.

But their behavior can be managed with medication and treatment.

CHAPTER THREE

HOW DOES ADHD AFFECT SOCIETY?

The 2016 National Survey of Children's Health (NSCH) showed that about 6.1 million US children have ADHD. ADHD also affects 10 million US adults. Many people with ADHD are teenagers. Studies show that 5.9 to 7.1 percent of teens have been diagnosed with ADHD.

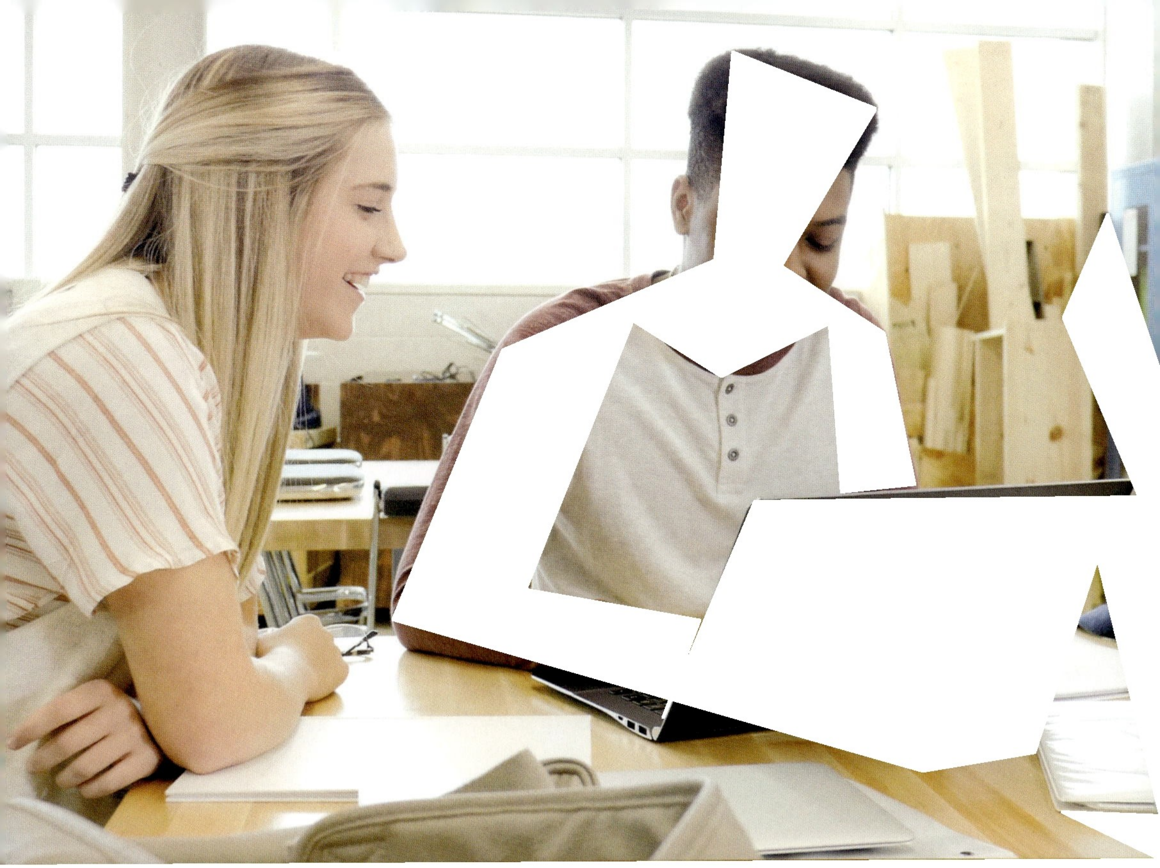

Gender can influence the type of symptoms a person with ADHD experiences.

ADHD affects people of all ages, races, and genders. But not all groups of people are diagnosed at the same rate. ADHD symptoms appear differently in boys and girls. Rates vary across races too.

ADHD AND GENDER

A 2012 analysis compared ADHD rates between males and females. It found that males are more than twice as likely to be diagnosed with ADHD. Females were three times less likely to have the hyperactive-impulsive type.

Women and girls are less likely to be diagnosed with ADHD. Their symptoms may be less obvious. Sometimes the signs are overlooked. This can lead to missed diagnoses. "Girls are not as hyperactive," says Dr. Patricia Quinn. She is the director and cofounder of the National Resource

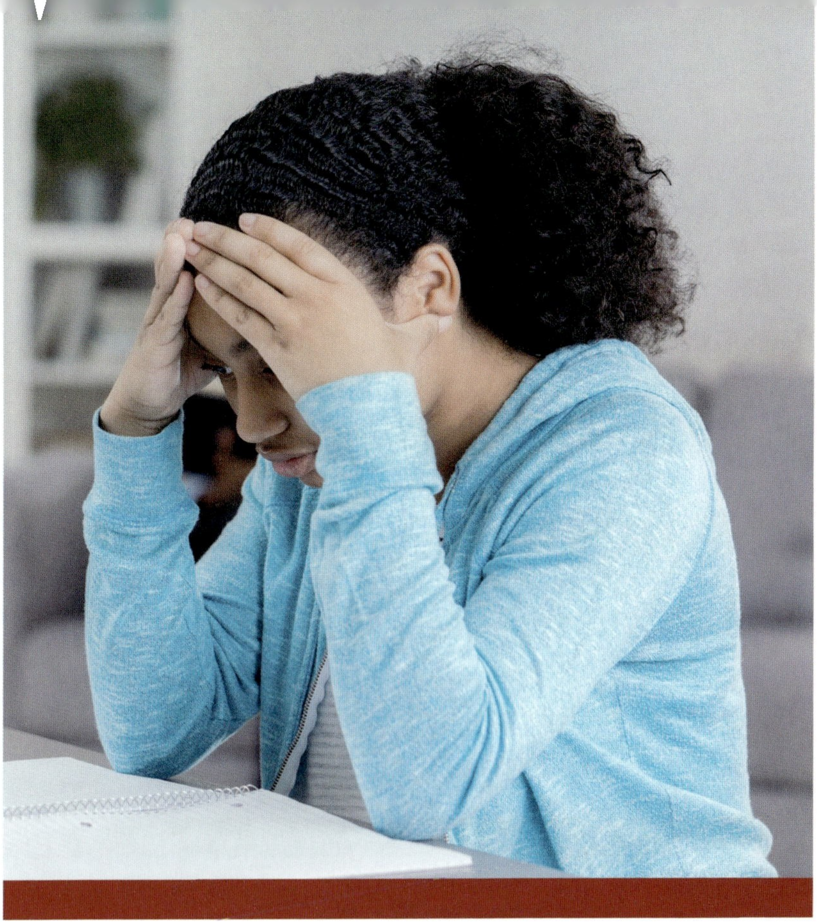

ADHD symptoms in girls may be harder to recognize.

Center for Girls and Women with ADHD. "People imagine little boys bouncing off the walls. [They] think: That's what ADHD looks like."[4] A girl may have ADHD but not show this behavior.

Untreated ADHD can lead to other mental health problems such as anxiety or depression. People with undiagnosed ADHD do not receive the proper support to help them succeed. This can damage self-esteem and harm mental health.

GIRLS AND INATTENTION

Andrea Burns has inattentive ADHD. She showed symptoms in middle school but never went to a doctor. She almost failed out of college. One of her professors suggested she get tested for ADHD. She was diagnosed with the inattentive kind of ADHD and given medication. It helped right away. She said, "For the first time I felt in control in the classroom."

Quoted in Maureen Connolly, "ADHD in Girls: Why It's Ignored, Why That's Dangerous," ADDitude, *October 2, 2019. www.additudemag.com.*

ADHD AND RACE

Studies show differences in ADHD diagnosis rates across racial groups. NSCH found that 8.4 percent of white parents had a child with ADHD. More than 10 percent of Black parents had a child with ADHD. Only 6 percent of Hispanic/Latino parents reported having a child with ADHD.

Scientists continue to study how race and ADHD interact. A 2017 study found that Black youth were more likely to be diagnosed with ADHD than white children. Other studies report that Hispanic children are less likely to have an ADHD diagnosis

PERCENTAGE OF US CHILDREN DIAGNOSED WITH ADHD OR A LEARNING DISABILITY

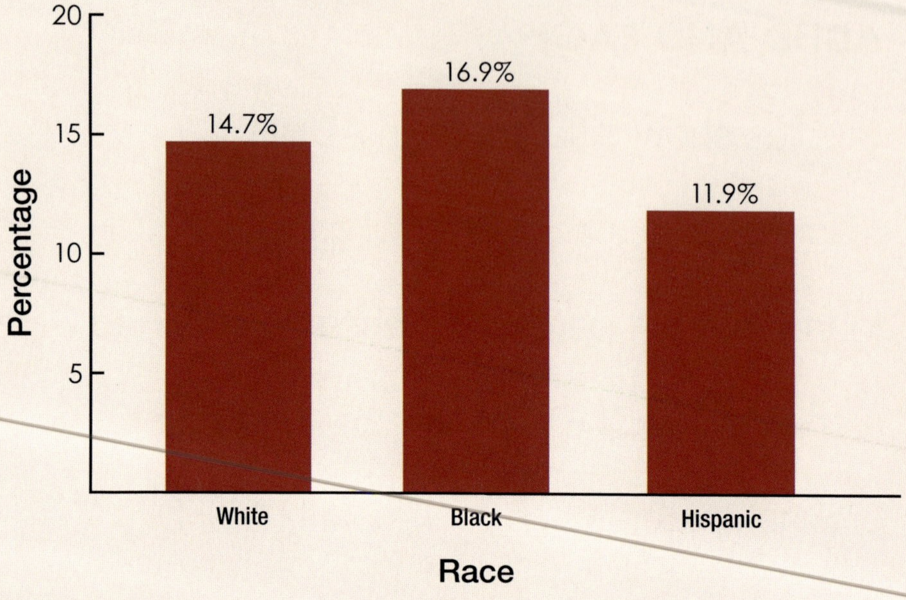

Source: Benjamin Zablotsky and Josephine M. Alford, "Racial and Ethnic Differences in the Prevalence of Attention-Deficit/Hyperactivity Disorder and Learning Disabilities Among US Children Aged 3–17 Years," CDC, March 2020. www.cdc.gov.

Black youth are more likely to have an ADHD or learning disability diagnosis than white or Hispanic youth.

than white children. This does not mean they are less likely to develop ADHD. Doctors may miss diagnoses. These children may not have seen a doctor for their behavior.

Evidence also shows that Black and Latino youth are less likely to get ADHD treatment. There are a few reasons for this. Some doctors have **racial bias** when treating their patients. They may be unaware of their bias. Doctors may treat patients differently based on their race. Some minority families feel that doctors do not take their concerns seriously. Another reason is a lack of trust. Some racial groups have less faith in doctors. They may have had bad experiences with doctors in

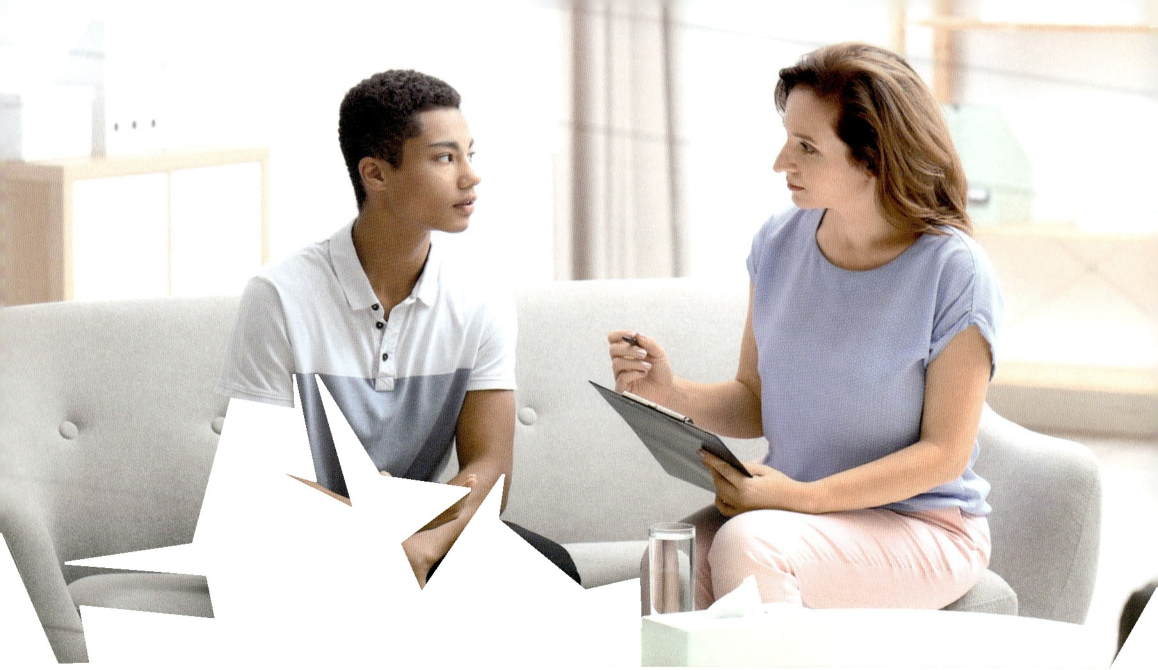

Some minority families have had bad experiences with doctors and psychologists. This may make them less likely to seek medical help.

the past. These groups are less likely to seek medical help. They choose to deal with issues like homework difficulties or forgetfulness at home.

A 2016 study found that children of color with ADHD were less likely to take ADHD medicine. Just 36 percent of Black kids and

30 percent of Latino kids with ADHD took medication. In comparison, 65 percent of white children with ADHD took medication.

ADHD AT SCHOOL AND WORK

ADHD can impact performance at work and in school. For example, children might get sent to the principal's office for disruptive behavior. They may have difficulty following directions. This can result in getting lower grades than they are capable of.

According to CHADD, 32 percent of students with the combined type of ADHD drop out of high school. Just 15 percent of teens without a mental disorder drop out.

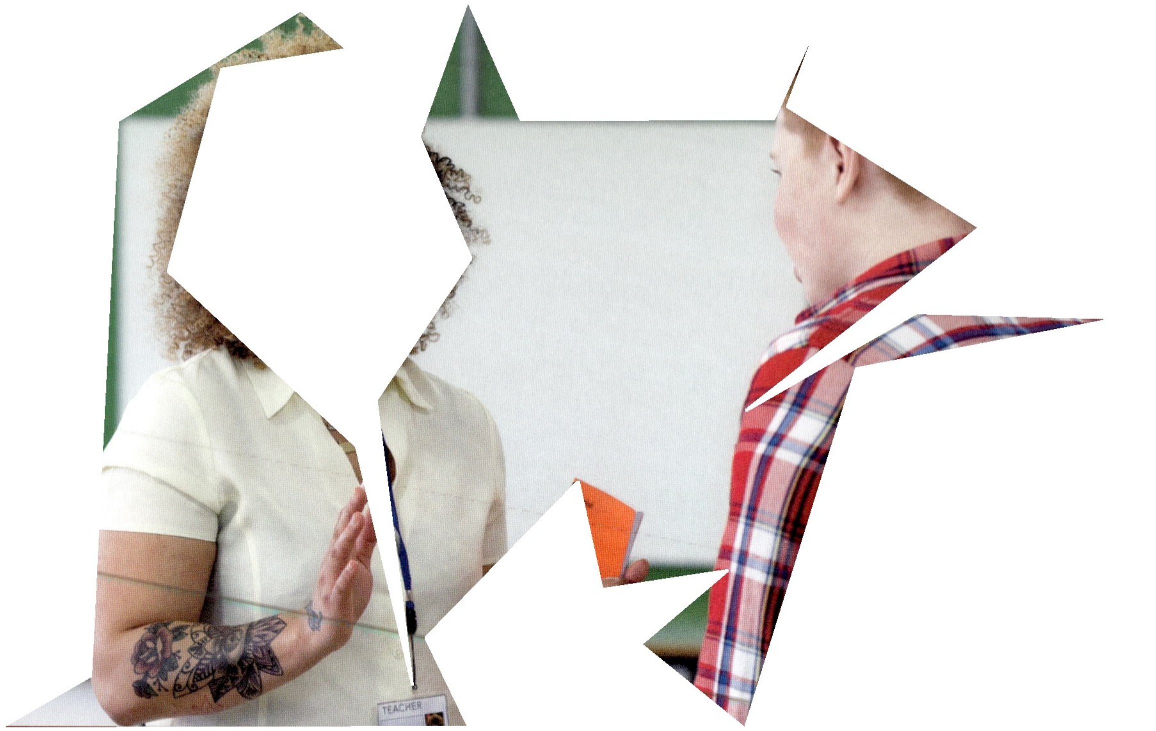

Untreated ADHD can lead to behaviors that cause problems at school.

Another study found that teens with ADHD are less likely to attend a four-year college. Those who do go to college may find it hard to succeed.

Lack of focus can cause problems at work too. Sitting through long meetings can be tough. Time management can be a challenge.

These obstacles don't mean that people with ADHD are doomed to fail. There are laws to help people with ADHD. The Individuals with Disabilities Education Act requires schools to help kids with ADHD. Teachers may give these students extra time on tests. Teachers can also help by keeping a schedule. They set clear expectations. Scheduling breaks is helpful. This can include time to move around or be outside. "Even something as simple as letting them go get a drink of water . . . can

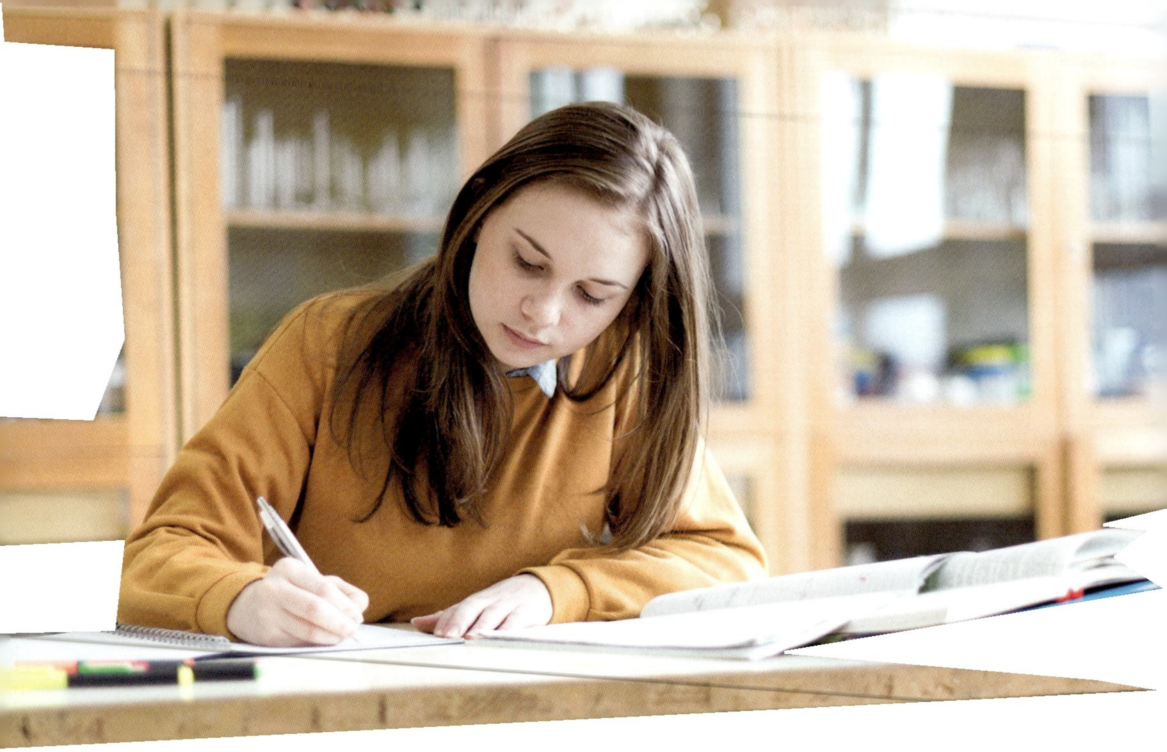

A student with ADHD may be given extra time to complete a test.

provide a moment of activity," says clinical scientist Keath Low.[5]

Family members can offer support too. Experts say sticking to a daily routine is key. Parents can help their child create a schedule. They can reward good behavior.

It's important to stay educated on how to manage ADHD. "ADHD touches everybody in the family in a daily, significant way," says Dr. Edward Hallowell. "Let each member of the family become a part of the solution."[6]

PARENT TO PARENT

There are many support groups for parents or guardians of kids with ADHD. One is Parent to Parent. It is run by CHADD. It has a series of eight online classes that help parents learn how to manage ADHD in the family. It features video lessons and downloadable resources. There are online chat rooms too. The classes are free. More information can be found on the CHADD website.

CHAPTER FOUR

HOW IS ADHD TREATED?

Living with ADHD can be frustrating. It can be especially hard for kids and teens. But leading a healthy and successful life is possible. ADHD can be managed with the right treatment. Each person responds differently to treatment.

Experts and patients work together to create a treatment plan. When the patient

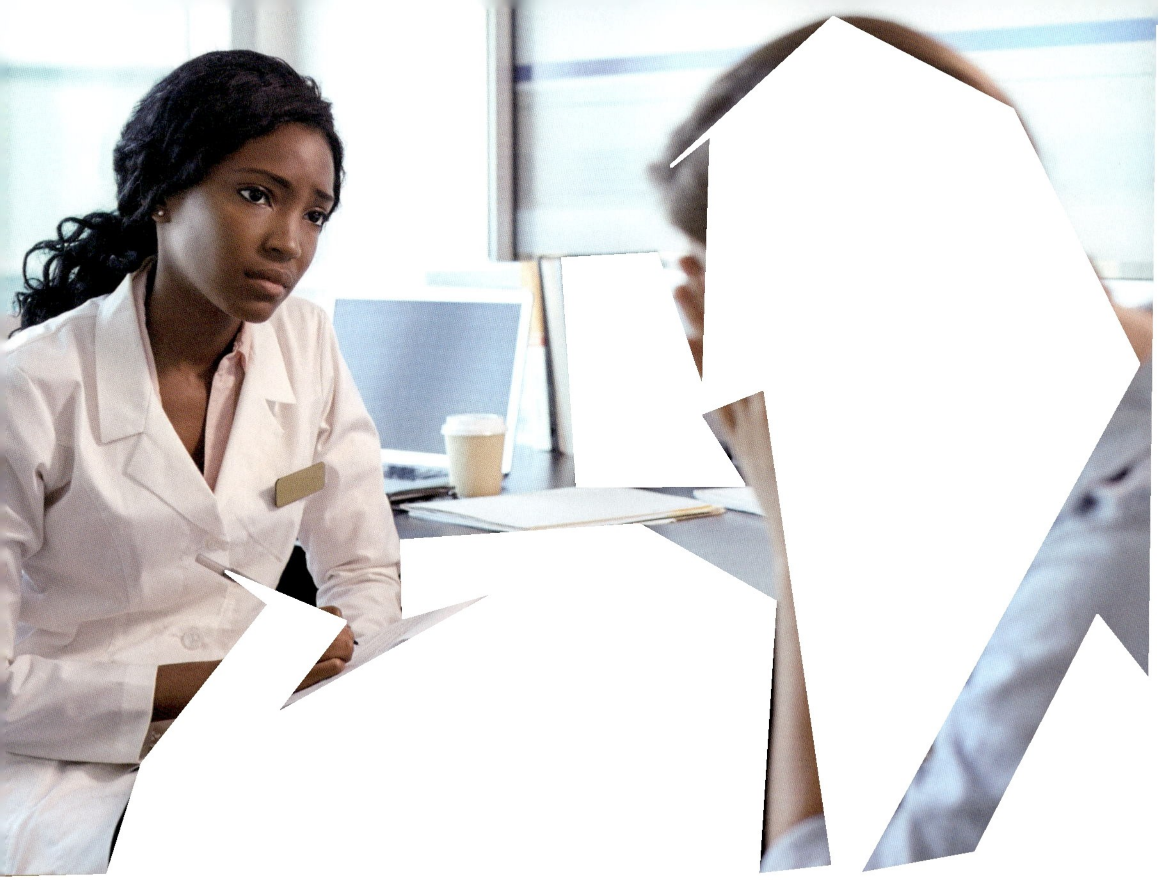

Developing an effective treatment plan may take patience.

is a child or teen, parents or guardians are also involved. Teachers can also help with the child's behavior at school. Finding the best ADHD treatment takes research and organization. It also requires patience when a drug or method doesn’t work. The treatment plan should be suitable for everyone involved. This includes the family members and teachers of a person with ADHD.

THERAPY

Therapy and medication are both used to treat ADHD. Most doctors recommend therapy before prescribing medication. Or they may recommend starting both at the same time. Cognitive behavioral therapy (CBT) helps patients replace unhealthy thoughts or actions with healthy ones. It teaches them how to create a routine.

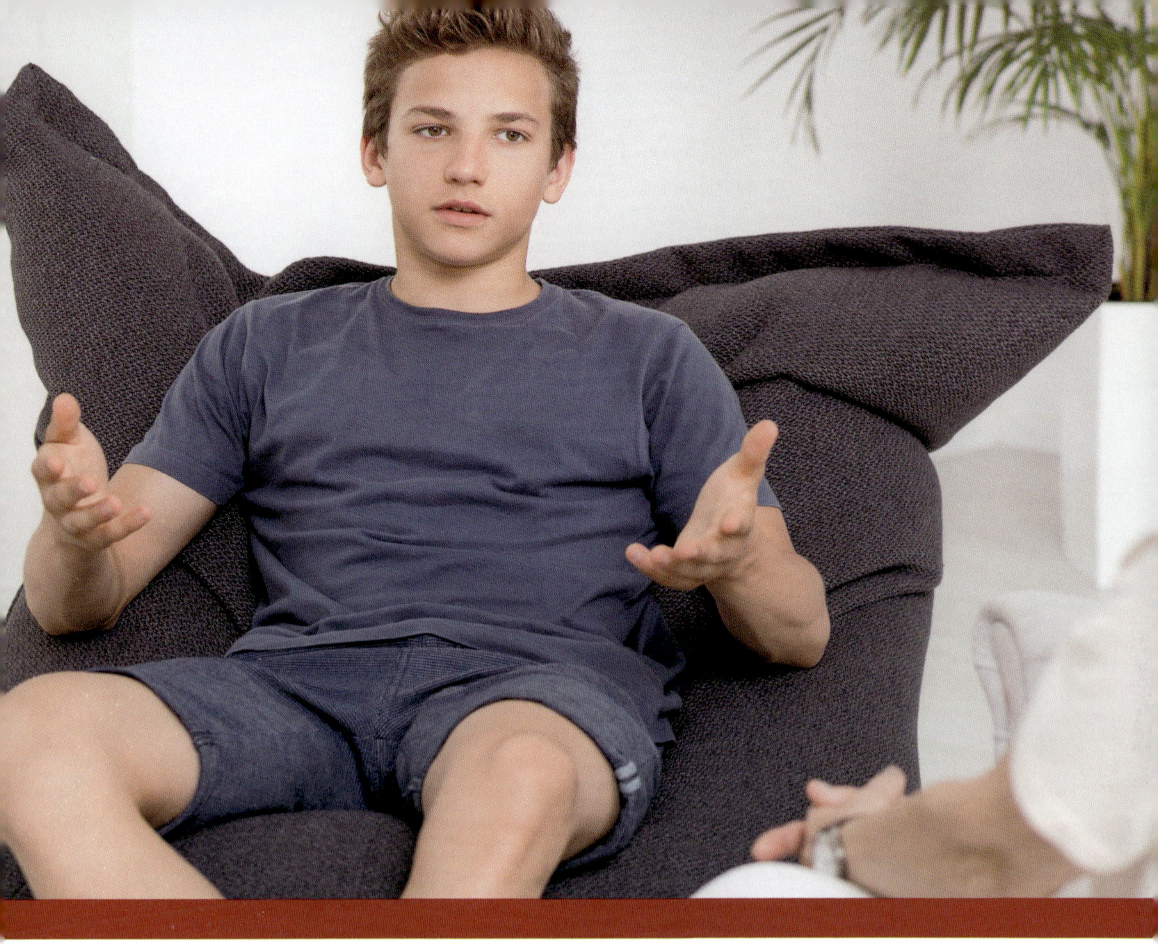

CBT helps patients with ADHD manage their symptoms.

In CBT sessions, ADHD patients talk with a trained counselor about how they are feeling. They discuss issues that are bothering them. They also explore negative behavioral patterns. Then the

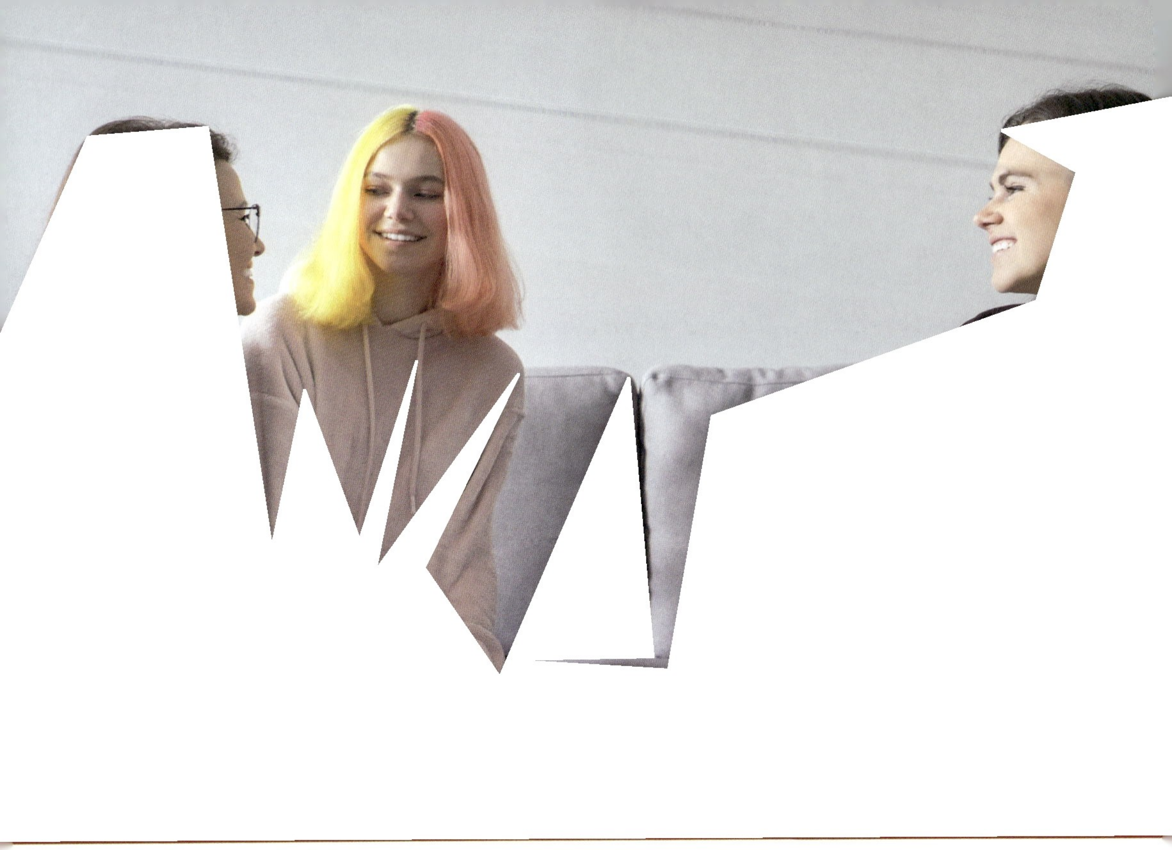

Psychologists may work with parents during therapy sessions.

counselor works with them to find healthier solutions. CBT for young children focuses on behaviors. The counselor may work with parents to develop a plan to improve behavior issues.

For example, a child might feel overwhelmed every time he sits down to do his homework. This may cause him to yell at his sister. Then he gets in trouble with his parents for the outburst. In this case, the counselor might suggest creating

SUMMER TREATMENT PROGRAMS

Summer Treatment Programs (STPs) are summer camps for youths with ADHD. Youths participate in fun activities and sports. STPs set clear expectations for their campers. Program leaders reward youths for their good behavior. They teach skills to manage ADHD symptoms. Parents or guardians also sign up for training classes at STPs. They learn skills that will help them manage their child's behavior at home. STPs take place in cities across the United States.

a checklist of his assignments before he begins. This way, he has a plan and won't lash out at others. A checklist can make goals seem more achievable. And having a clear set of steps can make tasks less overwhelming. This is especially helpful for children with ADHD.

CBT works especially well when it's combined with parent or guardian training. In these sessions, family members learn how to set rules and create daily routines to help the child thrive. They also learn what to do when problems arise. "You'll only set your child up for failure if you expect immediate and perfect results," says Dr. William Pelham Jr. "Instead, focus on rewarding small steps—and gradually work your way toward the desired outcome."[7]

Medication is not usually given to children under six. They are usually treated with just behavioral therapy. Parents receive training to manage their child's behavior. Kids ages

WHY EXERCISE HELPS

Exercise is important for staying fit and healthy. But it also helps with ADHD symptoms. Staying active is a natural way to boost norepinephrine levels. It increases focus and decreases hyperactivity. It also improves mood. Research has shown that exercise helps mental health. It can reduce stress and anxiety.

six and up often receive both therapy and medication. Treatment plans differ for each child. They vary depending on how serious the ADHD symptoms are.

MEDICATION

Psychiatrists prescribe medicine to ADHD patients. They most commonly prescribe stimulants to treat ADHD. These drugs increase the activity of the nervous system. They balance neurotransmitter levels in the brain.

Stimulants are either short acting or long acting. Short-acting stimulants are taken two or three times a day. They work within

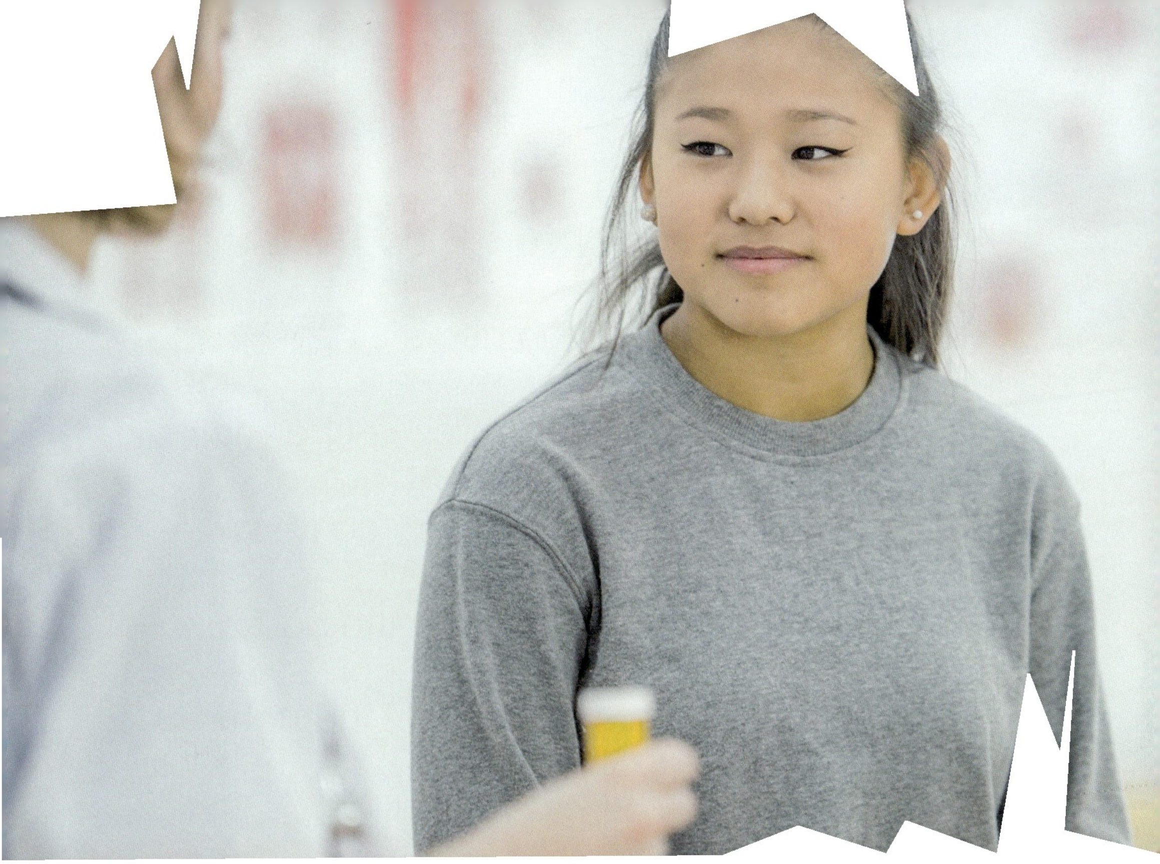

Medication is commonly prescribed to treat ADHD.

forty-five minutes. Their effects last from three to six hours. Long-acting stimulants are taken once a day. Most people take them in the morning. These drugs treat symptoms in phases. Part of the **dose** takes effect quickly. The rest of the dose starts working a few hours later. The effects last from eight to sixteen hours.

Stimulants are sold as pills, as chewable tablets, or in liquid form. Others come in the form of a patch to wear on the body. The medication enters the body through the skin.

The right dose varies from person to person. Doctors may need to adjust the dose so that it is more effective. They may change the dose as symptoms improve or worsen. Commonly prescribed stimulants include Ritalin and Adderall. Both can be short or long acting. About 70 to 80 percent

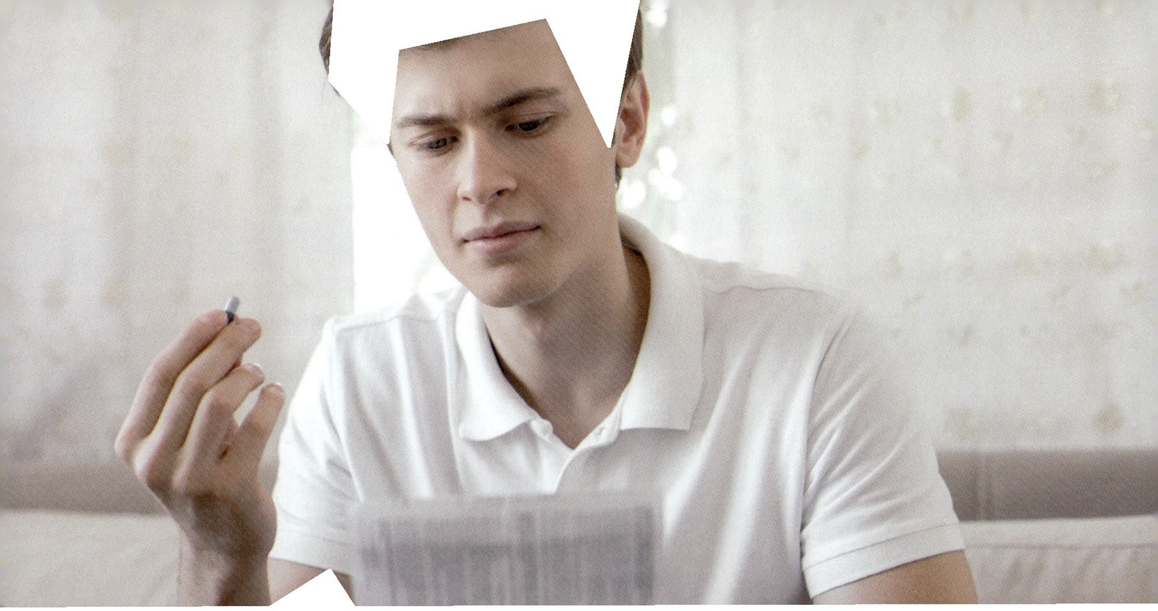

Medication should be taken only as prescribed.

of kids who have ADHD see improvements in behavior after taking these medications.

Stimulants may not have an effect for some people. Other patients may have a negative reaction to stimulants. They may be given different types of medication. These usually take longer to produce an effect. One example is Atomoxetine.

It works by increasing norepinephrine levels in the brain. Guanfacine was originally used to treat high blood pressure. It is also an ADHD medication. Some people take antidepressants to treat aspects of ADHD.

Of course, taking any drug can produce side effects. People often experience sleep disruption or headaches. An upset stomach and a decreased appetite are also common. Some people may experience anxiety.

It is important for anyone seeking ADHD treatment to discuss their options with a doctor. Most recommend a combination

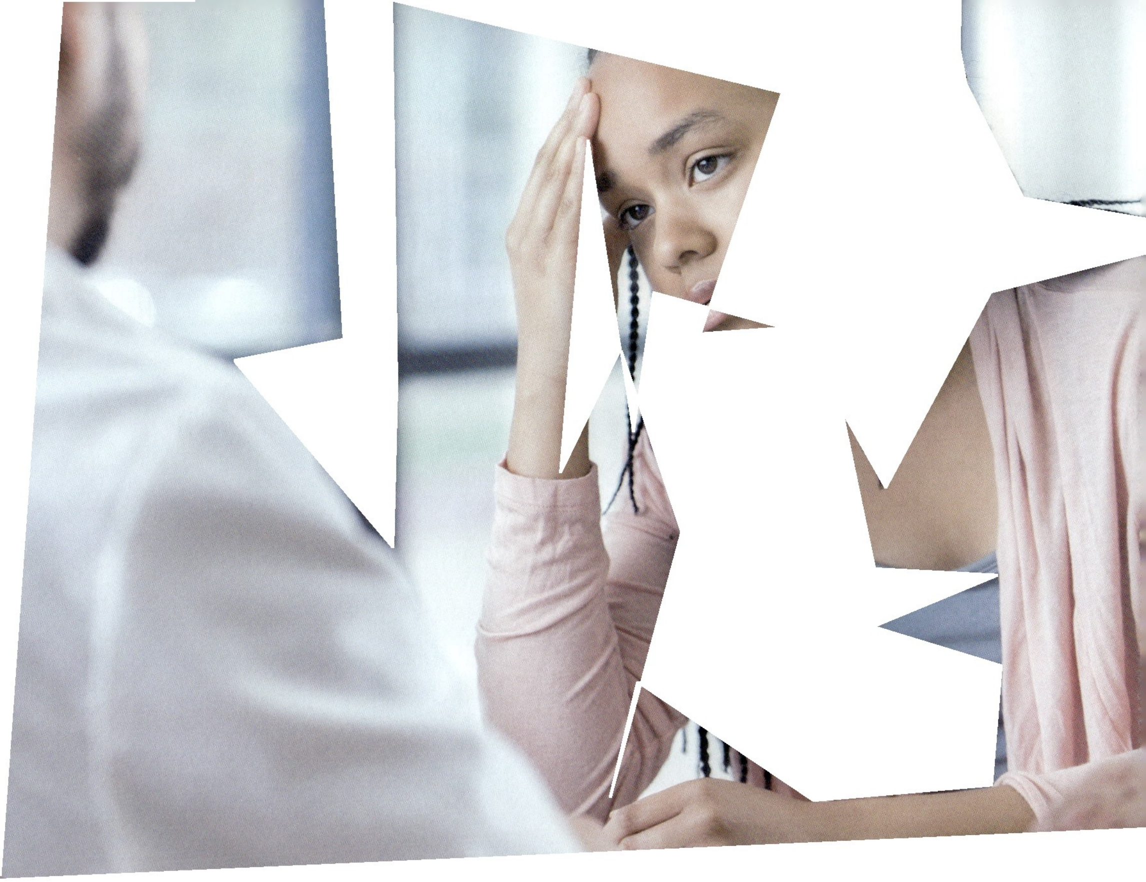

A patient should tell her doctor if she experiences any side effects from ADHD medication.

of therapy and medication. "If you've tried ADHD counseling . . . and didn't get the outcome you expected, try it again with medication," says Dr. William Dodson. "With medication, most people with ADHD are on a level playing field, often for the first time in their lives."[8]

POSITIVE OUTLOOK

ADHD is a lifelong condition. Some children who receive treatment no longer have serious symptoms by the time they are in their mid-twenties. It is possible to live a healthy and successful life with ADHD if the symptoms are managed properly.

Take Olympic shot-putter Michelle Carter. She grew up with ADHD. Paying attention at school was difficult. Reading and spelling were especially challenging.

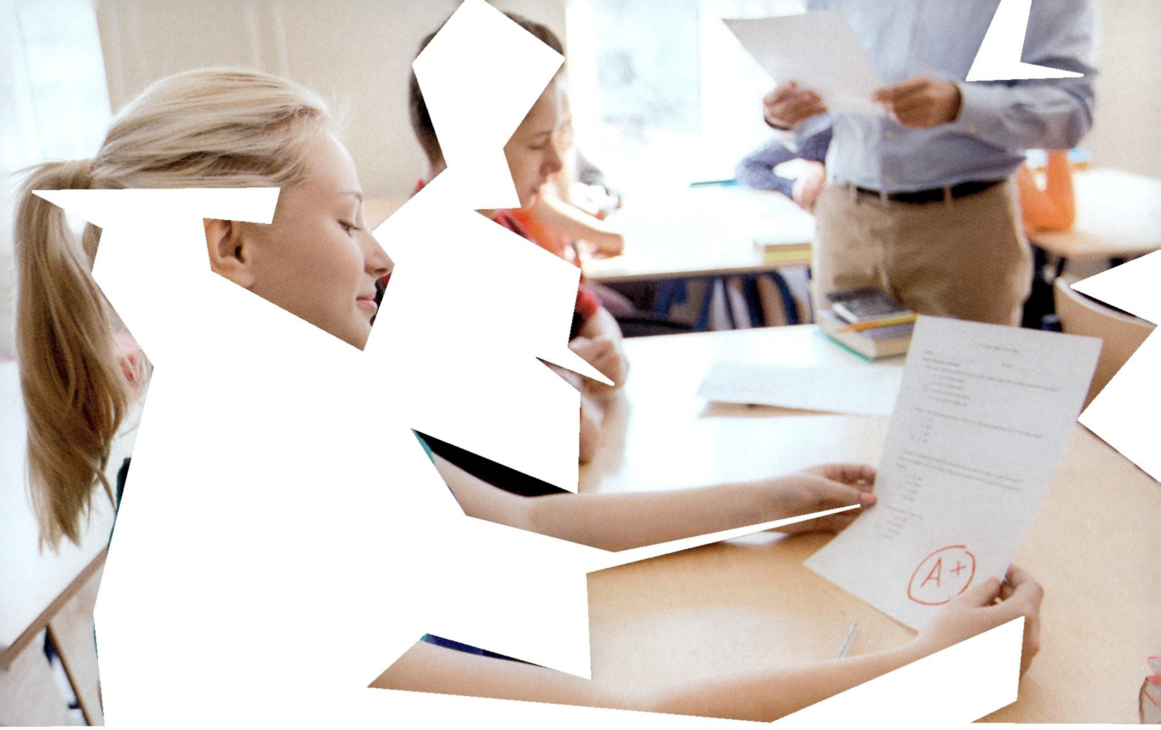

People with ADHD can find success when their symptoms are properly managed.

But with the support of her teachers and parents, Michelle learned the tools to help her succeed. Her teachers paid more attention to her in class. She also received tutoring four times a week. Slowly, her grades improved.

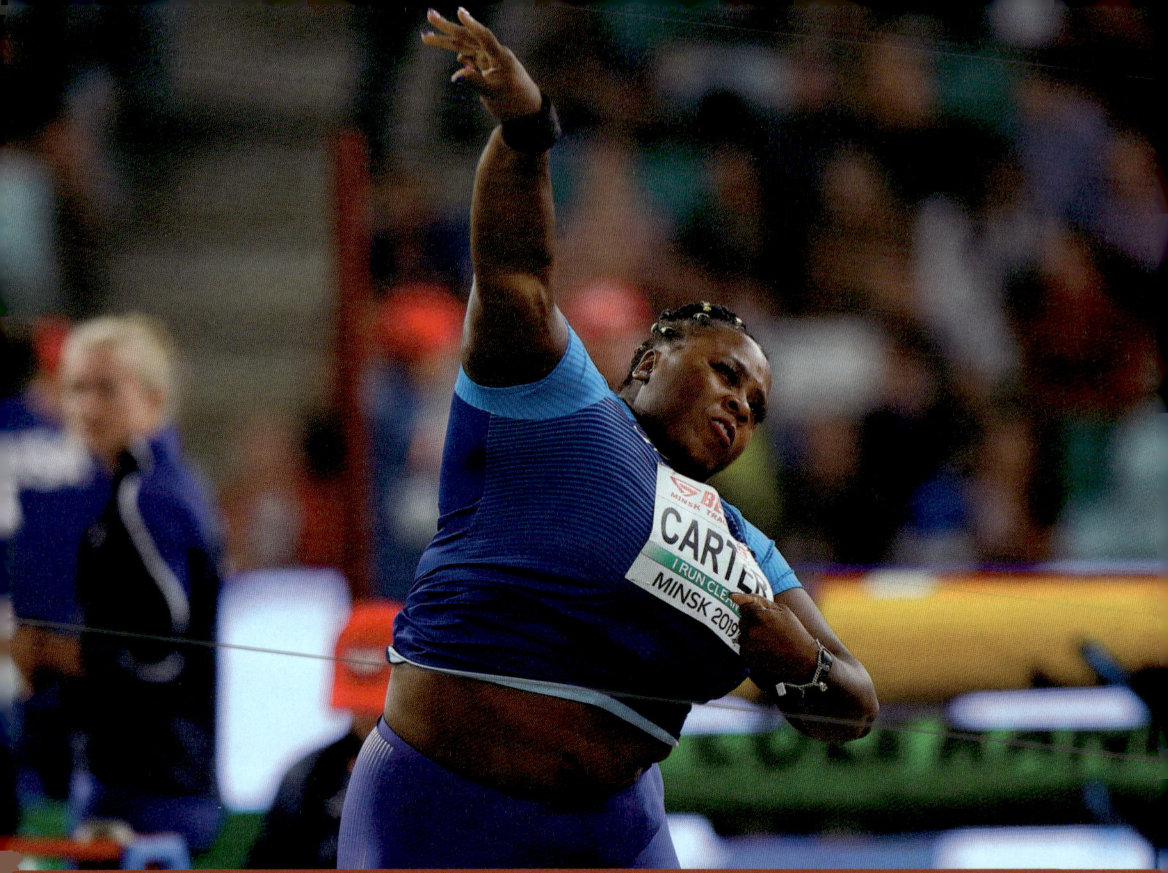

Michelle Carter is an Olympic shot-putter. She has spoken about her struggles with ADHD.

Michelle developed an interest in track and field. She especially enjoyed shot put. She created a daily exercise routine that gave her life structure. It also helped her stay in shape and channel her energy.

At fifteen, she made the US National Team. She made it to the Rio Olympic Games in 2016. She won a gold medal.

"They tell you as you get older [that] your learning issues will change or be different. No, I still struggle with those things today. . . . But I have to embrace that side of me," Carter says. "I don't care what anybody says. I think I'm awesome. I think I'm beautiful. I think I'm smart . . . I know that I am different. And I want everybody to feel that the way that they are is OK."[9]

dose

the amount of a drug or medication given at one time

hostile

unfriendly or aggressive

impulsive

inclined to act without thinking about consequences

pesticides

chemicals used to kill pests such as bugs and rats

psychiatrists

doctors who treat mental, emotional, or behavioral disorders

psychologist

a person who studies minds and behaviors

racial bias

prejudice against people of different races

symptoms

thoughts, behaviors, actions, or physical conditions that show a person has a disorder or disease

INTRODUCTION: AN OLYMPIC SUPERSTAR WITH GOLD-MEDAL FOCUS

1. Quoted in Aimee Crawford, "Bravo, Simone Biles, for Taking a Stand Against ADHD Stigma," *ESPN*, September 21, 2016. www.espn.com.

2. Quoted in Janice Rodden, "Having ADHD and Taking Medicine for It Is Nothing to Be Ashamed Of," *ADDitude*, September 14, 2016. www.additudemag.com.

CHAPTER ONE: WHAT IS ADHD?

3. Quoted in Caroline Miller, "ADHD and Behavior Problems," *Child Mind Institute*, 2021. https://childmind.org.

CHAPTER THREE: HOW DOES ADHD AFFECT SOCIETY?

4. Quoted in Rae Jacobson, "How Girls with ADHD Are Different," *Child Mind Institute*, 2021. https://childmind.org.

5. Keath Low, "8 Simple School Strategies for Students with ADHD," *Verywell Mind*, June 29, 2020. www.verywellmind.com.

6. Edward Hallowell, "12 Ways to Build Strong ADHD Families," *ADDitude*, June 19, 2019. www.additudemag.com.

CHAPTER FOUR: HOW IS ADHD TREATED?

7. Quoted in "'None of Us Were Trained How to Be Good Parents,'" *ADDitude*, October 11, 2019. www.additudemag.com.

8. William Dodson, "ADHD's Common Denominators," *ADDitude*, May 7, 2020. www.additudemag.com.

9. Quoted in "Video: Michelle Carter Wins Olympic Gold with Dyslexia and ADHD," *Understood*, 2021. www.understood.org.

BOOKS

Melissa Abramovitz, *Kids and ADHD.* San Diego, CA: ReferencePoint Press, 2018.

Carla Mooney, *Teens and ADHD*. San Diego, CA: ReferencePoint Press, 2017.

Allison Tyler, *Thriving with ADHD: Workbook for Teens*. Emeryville, CA: Rockridge Press, 2020.

INTERNET SOURCES

Traci Angel, "Everything You Need to Know About ADHD," *Healthline*, September 5, 2020. www.healthline.com.

"Attention Deficit Hyperactivity Disorder," *National Institute of Mental Health*, September 2019. www.nimh.nih.gov.

"Attention Deficit Hyperactivity Disorder (ADHD)," *CDC*, n.d. www.cdc.gov.

"Attention Deficit Hyperactivity Disorder (ADHD) in Children," *Mayo Clinic*, June 25, 2019. www.mayoclinic.org.

WEBSITES

ADDitudeMag.com and ADDitude Magazine
www.additudemag.com

This site and quarterly publication contain information, statistics, and articles about ADHD.

Child Mind Institute
https://childmind.org

This site contains information about children struggling with mental health and learning disorders.

Children and Adults with Attention Deficit Hyperactivity Disorder (CHADD)
https://chadd.org

This site contains resources about ADHD for kids, teens, and parents.

Cover: © fizkes/iStockphoto
5: © Nikada/iStockphoto
7: © Leonard Zhukovsky/
Shutterstock Images
9: © Brian/iStockphoto
11: © VH-studio/Shutterstock Images
13: © SDI Productions/iStockphoto
16: © Constantinis/iStockphoto
18: © SolStock/iStockphoto
20: © fizkes/Shutterstock Images
24: © yak62/iStockphoto
27: © Tomwang112/iStockphoto
28: © cheapbooks/
Shutterstock Images
30: © photosaint/iStockphoto
32: © PR Image Factory/
Shutterstock Images
35: © RoBeDeRo/iStockphoto
37: © Chainarong Prasertthai/
iStockphoto
41: © Daisy-Daisy/iStockphoto
43: © SDI Productions/iStockphoto
45: © SDI Productions/iStockphoto
48: © Red Line Editorial
50: © New Africa/Shutterstock Images
52: © DGLimages/iStockphoto
54: © AndreaObzerova/iStockphoto
57: © monkeybusinessimages/
iStockphoto
59: © KatarzynaBialasiewicz/
iStockphoto
60: © Valeriy_G/iStockphoto
65: © FatCamera/iStockphoto
67: © bymuratdeniz/iStockphoto
69: © SDI Productions/iStockphoto
71: © Syda Productions/
Shutterstock Images
72: © Andrew Makedonski/
Shutterstock Images

Doris Edwards has been a writer and educator for more than twenty years. She has written dozens of articles and books for young readers on a variety of topics, including historical and current events, health and mental health disorders, and money management and careers. Edwards lives in New York City with her husband and Siamese cat.